The Art of Human Care

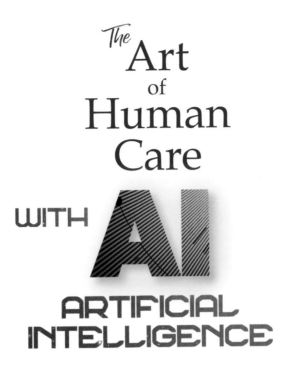

WITH AI

ARTIFICIAL INTELLIGENCE

HASSAN A. TETTEH

Inquiries about this book should be addressed to:
TCG Publishing
Bethesda, Maryland, USA
(800) 838-7061

www.doctortetteh.com

The Art of Human Care with AI
Hassan A. Tetteh
ISBN: 978-1-7336654-4-5
Library of Congress Control Number: 2020920150

Written by Hassan A. Tetteh
Cover Design by Karen McDiarmid | Book Design by Karen McDiarmid
Illustrated by Rose Freeman

Printed in Canada

10 9 8 7 6 5 4 3 2 1

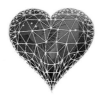

For
all who introduce
a new order of things
for good

There is nothing more difficult to take in hand,
more perilous to conduct, or more uncertain in its success,
than to take the lead in the introduction of
a new order of things.

—*Niccolo Machiavelli*

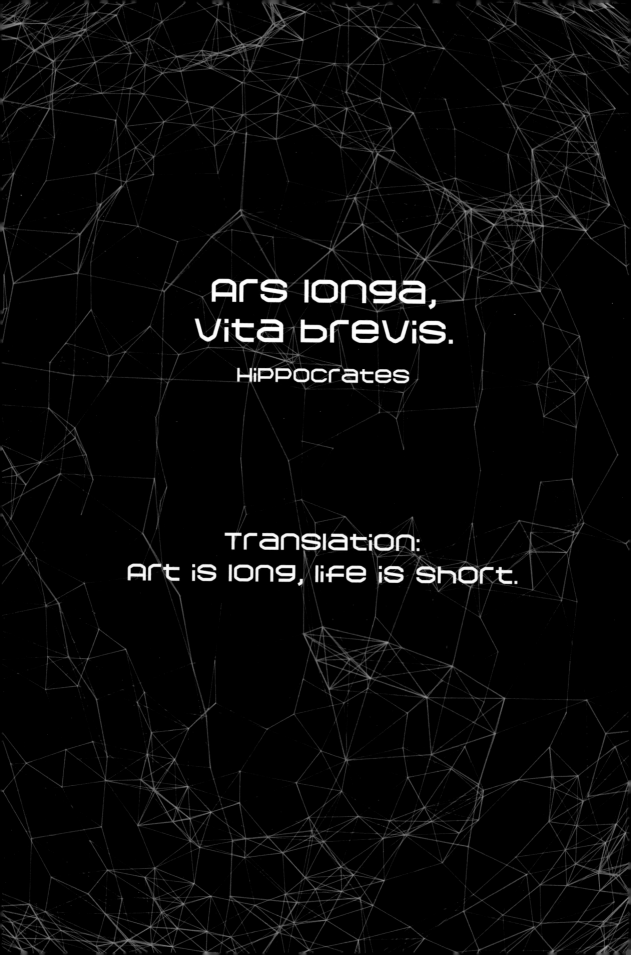

Ars longa,
Vita brevis.

Hippocrates

Translation:
Art is long, life is short.

contents

Foreword

Colonel (Ret.) Stoney Trent, Ph.D.

President, The Bulls Run Group (A Human-Machine Systems Company)

In 2018, the Honorable Dana Deasy, the Department of Defense (DoD) Chief Information Officer, asked me to plan the establishment of the Joint Artificial Intelligence Center (JAIC). Mr. Deasy's vision was for this center to lead the transformation of the world's largest bureaucracy with and for artificial intelligence. He had come to the DoD from the finance industry where banks had evolved over the past 20 years from companies that used information technology to information technology companies that execute financial transactions. Similarly, the DoD would require a deliberate, sustained investment to retool its workforce, systems, and processes—or people, technology and work.

Successful innovations happen at the intersection of people, technology, and work. Failed innovations attempt to separate this "innovation triad," envisioning one element as a replacement for another. History and science have demonstrated how technology never replaces people. Rather it changes the nature of work and creates new roles and unintended consequences. Therefore, leading transformation with artificial intelligence requires deliberate investments toward understanding the innovation triad.

To transform the DoD, the JAIC needed to reach and impact the myriad of communities that comprise the department. One community that impacts the readiness of all others is the military healthcare community. To affect this community, I sought a passionate work domain expert that could grant immediate credibility to the change initiative—someone to spark a brushfire of change in military medicine. Dr. Tetteh fit that model.

In *The Art of Human Care with AI*, Dr. Tetteh advocates for improving health by treating patients as people, rather than objects. Healthcare is technology-enabled and human-centric. One of Dr. Tetteh's salient points in this book, "never engineer the human out," has been validated through decades of resilient systems engineering research and practice. Humans are the source of resilience in any system. As humans, we are irreplaceable sources of adaptation, sense making, goal setting, and empathy. We make and use technology to achieve our desired outcomes. And we reject technologies when they confuse, complicate, or hamper our work.

AI doesn't just happen, and there is no "off-the-shelf" AI. Technologists require knowledge about the realities of the people and work they intend to impact. AI successes in low risk, everyday settings, e.g., internet search algorithms, video games, or product recommenders, happen because technologists have access to the people and work they are trying to support. Unfortunately, high risk work domains, like healthcare, are closed to most technologists. They lack access to workplaces, workers, data, and legacy systems that impact the performance of new technologies. Consequently, innovations require expert boundary spanners who understand the work domain and can translate facts about people and work into artifacts to inform technology development. Dr. Tetteh's health mission in the Joint AI Center provided such a bridge.

The Art of Human Care with AI offers an inspirational vision for a future of healthcare fully enabled with AI. It is not a future that will materialize simply at the hands of a computer or data scientist. It is a future that will emerge from collaboration, openness, vision, and hard work. Dr. Tetteh has gathered us around a campfire, sharing his stories while striking flint over the kindling. I pray his spark begets the intended brushfire—for the betterment of humanity.

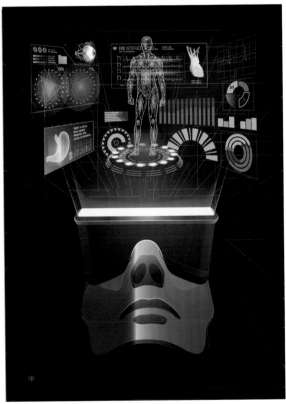

Rose Freeman

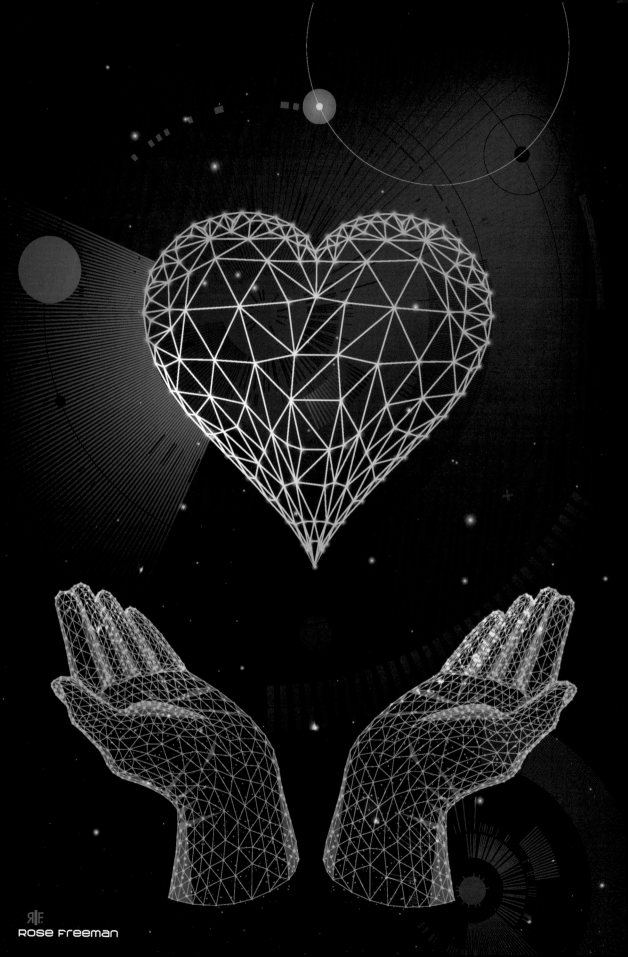

ROSE FREEMAN

Introduction

Hassan A. Tetteh

When you picked up this book and looked at the title on the cover, you might have wondered, "What does artificial intelligence (AI) have to do with *The Art of Human Care*? When you think of AI, blockbuster movies such as *The Terminator* and *Bladerunner* that portray dystopian futures may come to mind. When you think about AI assisting your doctor or nurse, you might recoil and think, "I don't want this technology to be calling the shots when it comes to my health." But the truth is that this technology has been helping people heal and live better lives for millennia. AI should be regarded as one more tool to help us deliver healthcare better.

AI offers a tremendous amount of potential in healthcare. To develop AI is to train a machine to scale and apply data (information). That's why AI has value for healthcare—it provides a lot of data and a lot of information on people. AI streamlines all the information and gives healthcare workers the ability to do a great amount of good.

If you interviewed me when I graduated from medical school in 1998 and asked, "Dr. Tetteh, what are you going to be doing in 22 years?" I'd have probably replied, "General surgery. I'm going to be a general surgeon." But that's not what I'm doing right now. I would never have thought that I would be doing what I am doing today.

A little while back, I was invited to present the opening keynote speech for the American Medical Informatics Association. Why is a cardiothoracic surgeon doing the opening keynote for the American Medical Informatics Association?

Well, it's because I realized years ago that there's something about these computers and technology that's impacting medicine. So, I set out to learn a little bit about it. Before I had gotten very far into this inquiry, I said, "Holy Christmas! There's something called informatics."

Informatics applies computer programming, mathematics, and statistics to improve outcomes in any number of disciplines, including medicine. I didn't even know that clinical informatics was a medical specialty. Then a few years ago, I discovered that there was a board certification for informatics. I wondered, "How do I get into that?" I became obsessed with learning more.

I discovered a clinical pathway to this certification for physicians with experience working in the field. Fortunately, throughout my career, I had worked in many roles as a clinical informaticist and concentrated my studies in gaining formal training as well. I initially thought the requirements would be something futuristic or sci-fi. The principle of applying clinical informatics to deliver better care just made sense. "This is amazing," I said to myself. "I am going to pursue this." So, that's what I did.

Informatics is really something we've been doing all along. It is using information and technology to help us do our jobs better. Even if unknowingly, we have been utilizing this as physicians, as nurses, as practitioners in health. We take information and use technology to help deliver care.

When I was at the National War College, my background in informatics led me to an opportunity to study AI. I was seeing AI everywhere. I thought, "This is like electricity when it was first introduced. AI is the electricity of today. This is going to be great." But it took an evolution of understanding and personalizing to realize, "Hey, this innovation is all about trying to find the right solutions to the right problems at the right time."

First of all, we can integrate AI into some of our diagnostic tools. For example, machines trained to read X-rays can point out abnormalities more accurately than the naked eye and spend a lot less time doing so. And in Europe and India, law enforcement is working hand-in-hand with Facebook, deploying algorithms to identify people at risk for suicide.

We should look at AI as a way to use information and technology to help us do our work better. Partnering with AI, we will be able to do human care—plus find purpose in, personalize, and form partneships in our care—in an even more robust and accurate way. Now, we can do precision medicine by basing our treatment on the individual's genetic makeup. Instead of just saying, "Hey this happened to a middle-aged man who has this particular problem," we'll be able to be a lot more specific. We'll be able to determine our diagnosis from information gathered at the genomic and microscopic level. That precise information will guide us in how we treat a patient and which medicines we administer.

Again, the purpose is to deliver good care, better care, by utilizing all the tools available. Wouldn't it be cool if, like in *Star Trek*, we had the little machine that could scan the body for information instead of guessing about things? We would come up with a more accurate diagnosis to help prevent disease, cure disease, or provide treatment more effectively.

AI has that potential. It can be that tool that helps us deliver healthcare better. However, in the final analysis, we need to keep humans center and present. And so, I give you *The Art of Human Care with AI*.

AI Changing Lives

PARTNERSHIPS CREATING ART

"Wherever the art of medicine is loved, there is also a love of humanity."
—Hippocrates

Many computer systems already generate creative output, such as 3D illustrations, that could be considered art. Produced with mathematical formulas and algorithms, AI artwork requires programmers, computers, and artists working together to generate art.

Human Care Theory

•••••• DR. HASSAN A. TETTEH, M.D.

WHAT is Human Care? •••• Human Care is timely, comprehensive care that advances each person's total health in body, mind, and spirit.

WHAT problems does Human Care address? •••• Human Care challenges the current system that is not patient-centered and that is perpetuating fragmented care, escalating costs, and inefficient delivery.

WHY is Human Care important? •••• Human Care produces a healthier society by meeting the patient's need for real care, the physician's desire to be a true healer, and the country's desire for actual value for dollars spent on healthcare.

PURPOSE •••• Revive Your Healing Passion
Resurrect your commitment to the honorable and meaningful purpose of helping people feel better.

Realize Your Healing Power
Grasp the impact you make as you restore people's health so they can realize their purpose and continue the chain reaction of changing the world.

PERSONALIZATION •••• Discover Your Patient's Present
Learn your patient's current state of being, including his or her values, dreams, and gifts for the world.

Maximize Your Patient Encounters
Capitalize on each interaction to create trust and the respectful connection that can change the world.

PARTNERSHIP •••• Leverage Your Team Dream
Advance the collective care team effort to achieve a total health impact for all.

Shape Your Professional Horizon
Create your unique legacy to elevate and unify the healthcare community for a lasting impact on health and humanity.

CONCRETE RESULTS •••• • The antidote for burnout in healthcare.
• A new perspective on what it means to heal.
• A formula that delivers a new level of healing.
• The ideal model for providing effective care.
• A passion to make healthcare great again.

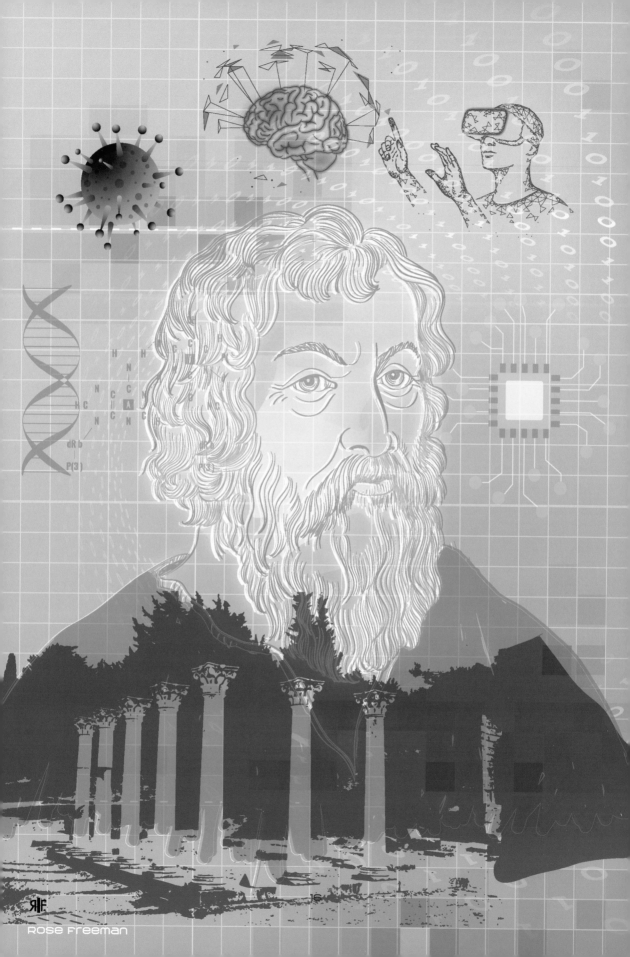

Chapter 1

AI and the History of Medicine

If you read my first two books in this series, *The Art of Human Care* and *The Art of Human Care and COVID-19*, you know that I like ancient history—especially the ancient history of Western medicine. Herophilus of Chalcedon, the physician to Alexander the Great, once admonished, "When health is absent, wisdom cannot reveal itself, art cannot become manifest, strength cannot fight, wealth becomes useless, and intelligence cannot be applied." Since human life began, our pursuit of health, whether our own or our loved ones', has transcended the pursuits of education, culture, and economics—and it always will.

Health is what's most important to us humans. Most of us can accomplish little without it. As Joseph Lister's work in antisepsis (handwashing) and Louis Pasteur's germ theory revolutionized medicine in the mid-nineteenth century, AI—artificial intelligence—will be this era's most important vehicle for improving healthcare.

I'm very excited about this new paradigm of healthcare technology. In simple terms, AI is computer-simulated intelligent human behavior. The Merriam Webster dictionary defines technology as "the practical application of knowledge, especially in a particular area."

The roots of Western medicine date back to ancient Greece. In *The Art of Human Care,* I wrote about Hippocrates and how he diagnosed and treated a middle-aged businessman's chest pain. Instead of subjecting him to the standardized treatments of the day, which involved snakes, dogs, food deprivation, and dream analysis, he took time to listen. In addition to prescribing treatment, he advised on healthy lifestyle choices. Today, we call Hippocrates "The Father of Medicine." New physicians, before they begin their practice, still take the Hippocratic oath.

It should be no surprise that our military is a leading force in integrating AI into healthcare today. Over the course of history, military medicine has time and time again made great advancements that have actually impacted civilian healthcare in a meaningful and robust way. Even if you only consider the short history of the United States of America, you will come up with many examples. In 1776, George Washington's Continental Army suffered from the scourge of smallpox to such a great extent that Washington mandated his soldiers to have inoculations to spurn the smallpox virus.

During the American Civil War, from 1861–1865, two recorded cases document that, for the first time, blood transfusion was used for treating bleeding following a leg amputation. During World War I, between the years 1914–1918, donor blood using citrate as a preservative-anticoagulant was introduced to save the lives of doughboys on the frontline. During this war, blood distribution was carefully coordinated, and specific indications for transfusion were established.

The use of transfusions to save lives quickly caught on in civilian medicine. By 1937, Cook County Hospital in Chicago, Illinois, established the first blood bank. In 1941, the United States entered World War II, and in 1942, the Army established the first military blood bank at the Walter Reed General Hospital. Despite early challenges, the program became the starting point for a much more massive initiative that would develop to save countless lives on and off the battlefield.

During the Vietnam War, from 1955–1973, and the first Gulf War, from 1990–1991, 24 percent of service members who were wounded in action died. Subsequent wars in Iraq and Afghanistan challenged our accepted concepts of trauma, resuscitation, and surgery. In those wars, over the course of the years 2003–2009, only 10 percent of service members who were wounded in action died. These lives were saved because of the novel utilization of blood transfusions and innovations in controlling bleeding.

Many influential military leaders have dedicated decades of work to shape the current military blood program into what it is today. The program continues to improve the way blood is collected, stored, shipped, and transfused in both military and civilian settings. The military's modernization and standardization of the blood program has served as a vanguard for best practices in critical medical therapy. When I was deployed during the Gulf War and the War in Afghanistan, we recognized how giving whole blood instead of a pack of red blood cells led to a better outcome in trauma injuries.

When I was a surgeon stationed on a U.S. Navy aircraft carrier, I often treated patients who had developed suspicious skin lesions from spending a great deal of time on deck in direct sunlight. It would often take weeks—sometimes months—before the ships reached port and I could transfer biopsies to pathologists for diagnosis. It was not uncommon for some of those lesions to come back as early cancers. You can imagine how that kind of time delay can impact the ability to treat a cancer case optimally. When I thought about this later, I realized that there's a lot of capability and a lot of potential use and application for how AI can be used to advance cancer diagnostics.

This technology isn't so abstract. In fact, one of my current roles is to promote the use of AI within the military's healthcare systems. Predictive health is one of nearly 30 projects I'm involved with through the Joint Artificial Intelligence Center's (JAIC's) Warfighter Health Mission Initiative. Predictive health, among other things, involves developing cancer-detecting AI applications that reduce the time it takes for cancer to be diagnosed so patients can be treated more quickly. The ultimate intent is that one day in the not-so-distant future, military healthcare providers in the field will be able to upload a medical image for analysis—or even analyze it on site—with AI algorithms that can examine the entire slide exhaustively, report if cancer is detected, and determine the type and stage of cancer.

Other areas where AI healthcare solutions are being innovated include analyzing health records, automating medical logistics, preventing suicide, and supporting point-of-injury treatment. As we pioneer more lifesaving and health-enhancing AI solutions for our troops, the rest of our nation—and the world—will benefit.

It turns out that this Hippocrates guy knew a little bit when he said, "He who wishes to be a surgeon should go to war." Not until I went to war, not until I saw those injuries, did I really know what he was talking about. My experiences during deployment led me to believe that AI has the potential to transform medicine as much or more than anesthesia, vaccines, antisepsis, or blood transfusions. We should regard AI as the tool that will help us deliver healthcare better—and make Hippocrates proud.

AI Changing Lives

AI and Cloud Computing Create Better Pharmaceuticals Faster

By combining cloud computing and AI, drug companies are developing drugs faster and with less expense. For example, Moderna employs a cloud-based computational capacity to run a variety of algorithms that design individual mRNA sequences to develop a new class of treatments using mRNA that uses instructions in DNA to build the proteins in human cells. These mRNA medicines tell the human body how to build certain proteins that treat or prevent an illness. Another drug company, Alphabet, uses AI to understand protein folding. When proteins get tangled and deformed, diseases such as diabetes, Parkinson's, and Alzheimer's can develop. Once the accurate protein structure models are compiled, researchers will be able to apply AI to develop drugs for these diseases more quickly.

THE ART OF HUMAN CARE
IN ACTION

HOW CAN
WE DO THIS BETTER?

Because I spent time at The War College and in a series of serendipitous events under many great mentors, I was given the opportunity to become the Chief of Warfighter Health. It has been an amazing experience! While at the National War College, I spent two years deep-diving into and researching AI. Yet, I learned more in a few months by practicing it—by using it and doing it every day—than I had in those two years. When you take theory and put it into practice, incredible things happen.

We are advancing five categories of AI at the JAIC: health records analysis, medical imagery classification, automated medical logistics, suicide prevention, and point of injury treatment support. The theory behind our work at the JAIC is a novel one. We aren't developing technology in a vacuum and then forcing it on professionals. Instead, we are developing the technology alongside the professionals. At the JAIC, there are professionals working alongside data scientist engineers to collaborate and build solutions for the problems we've identified. And I have brought my crazy philosophy of human care—purpose, personalization, and partnerships—to this practice. There is a magic that's happening.

A few weeks ago, I was in the operating room, and something happened that illustrates why it is so pivotal to have practitioners develop AI solutions alongside technology professionals. In the field, we have the perspective and the inclination to see what is working and what won't work. In this case, the liver surgeon was taking a biopsy of a liver we had recovered for transplant. We happened to be at a small hospital, so we had to wait for the pathologist to give us a reading that showed the amount of necrosis and fat in the cells. That would tell us whether the liver could be used for transplant. We waited for four hours because the pathologist was out, and they had to bring in the technician. It was ridiculous. While I was there waiting, I thought about informatics and AI— like I always do. Really, what I was thinking about was how we could do this better.

At JAIC, we were working on medical imaging classification and delivering augmented reality microscopes trained to detect abnormalities (in this case, cancer). Through the microscope, I saw how it drew little rings around the abnormal cells. I turned to the other surgeon in the operating room and said, "What if we had that microscope here right now, snapped a picture, and sent it to the *pathologist? We wouldn't have to wait four hours and keep all these other transplant recipients waiting."*

Do you know what he said to me? "Bah, it'll never happen. I've been practicing surgery for 30 years. And I heard about this AI stuff 20 years ago."

Behind my mask, I had a big smile on my face. I recognized the challenge and realized that we have to be evangelists because our fellow practitioners may not know what the art of the possible is.

AI Changing Lives

A Purpose for AI: Early Pandemic Detection

It took nearly two years for scientists to pinpoint the probable source of the Ebola epidemic: a colony of Angolan free-tailed bats. Disease ecologist Barbara Han is using AI to predict these disease outbreaks—before they happen—by searching for the harbingers of outbreaks in the wild that eventually impact humans. Using computational models, she can sift through huge amounts of data to determine where the next potential pandemic might start. For example, she and her team trained a computer model to pick out new rodent species with high disease-carrying potential based on the traits they shared with 217 previously identified carriers of disease.

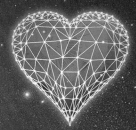

Part I

AI and Purpose

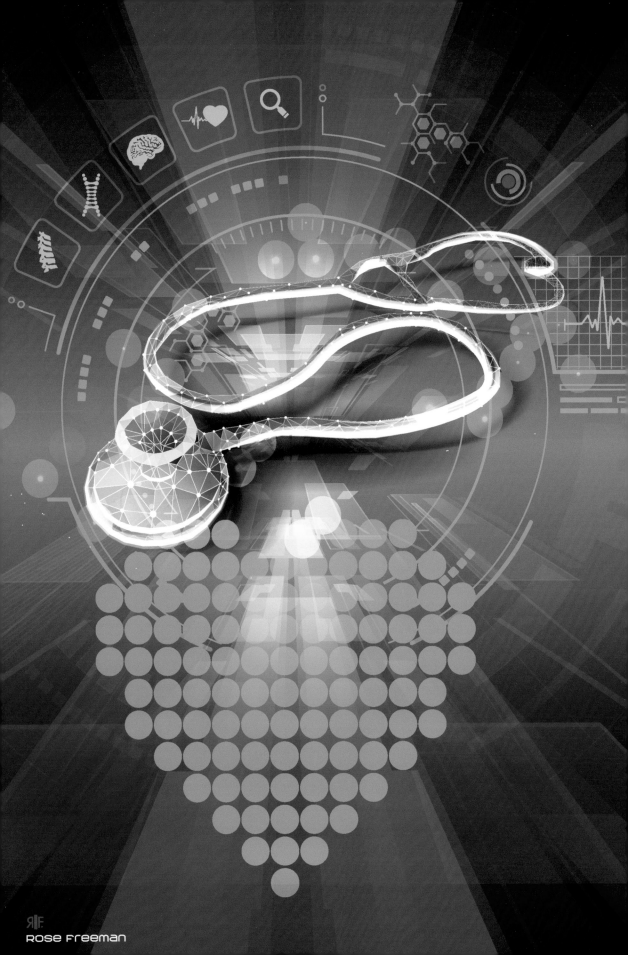

Chapter 2

The Purpose of AI and Why AI Is My Purpose

When we use AI to apply data science, algorithms, and advanced computer hardware to medical advancements, healthcare systems can advance health like never before. Instead of frustration with current unwieldy medical information systems, AI allows us to tap into the capabilities of smart devices and expand home-based care options such as telemedicine, which, due to the COVID-19 pandemic, is already in widespread use.

While computers that can learn and function exactly like the human mind are decades away, they are already beating real humans at strategy board games such as Go, guiding self-driving cars, and helping law enforcement with facial recognition. In medicine, an AI-enhanced voice interface could help pharmacists look up substitute drugs, provide tools to assist scheduling operating rooms and clinic appointments, and manage workflow efficiency in order to save time and human capital.

AI can direct more comprehensive personalized treatment plans and tailor treatments to each specific patient's needs and medical condition. Additionally, AI can help all providers care for injured, ill, and traumatized patients throughout the continuum of their recovery by providing a more precise picture of their condition. We can look to AI to inform clinical practice, interconnect clinicians and personalize care, and improve population health.

AI + EHR = Patient Centered Care

This might make me sound like a nerd, but I think the electronic health record (EHR) is a big-data breakthrough. Hundreds upon hundreds of scholarly articles tell us that EHRs have increased physicians' efficiency and decreased their burnout. In addition to providing an incredible amount of data along a patient's healthcare continuum, AI-augmented EHR can help decipher the meaning behind the data and help physicians accomplish their purpose in caring for an individual patient.

At Johns Hopkins Hospital in Baltimore, Maryland, an AI-powered "command center" receives data from throughout the medical center to make a real impact on individual patients' lives. Since the hospital invested in this particular AI enhancement, there has been a 60 percent increase in the hospital's ability to accept and care for complex cancer patients—60 percent! That's huge. In addition, patients admitted via the emergency room spent 25 percent less time in the ER before they were transferred to an inpatient unit. What thrilled me the most was that the hospital reduced operating room hold times by 60 percent. Overall, the investment in AI-leveraged technology has improved the hospital's efficiency and workflow tremendously—and that helps them meet their purpose of providing better patient care.

Another example is a rural hospital in southwest Michigan that invested in EHR in 2012. In 2016, the hospital enhanced the system with AI technology that used automated data entry and analyzed routine patient monitoring. The goal was to free up nurses' time. And it did. Nurses were able to spend more quality time caring for their patients. Additionally, an AI-driven early warning system built into the patient monitoring system reduced "code blues" by 56 percent. That means 56 percent less instances of patients going into cardiac or respiratory arrest thanks to consistent, AI monitoring. Because the AI identified subtle changes in the patients' vital signs and assigned risk scores, nurses were better informed on how to prioritize their patients' care.

The Fourth Industrial Revolution

At the 2016 World Economic Forum Meeting in Davos, the Fourth Industrial Revolution was defined as "the wave of technological advances that are changing the way we live, work, stay alive, and interact with each other and machines."

I don't believe for a minute that machines will take over the world and displace humans in the workplace or the hospital. AI enhances human skills, leading to more productive work. However, because the human brain is very complicated and still not entirely understood, certain essential activities will always remain uniquely human, for example, the ability to lead, empathize, create, and exercise judgment. Other activities have proved to be more efficiently performed by machines and artificial learning systems; for example, transactions (think ATMs), iterations (such as financial investments), and predictions (weather forecasts). A middle category of hybrid activities enlists humans and machines as symbiotic partners. Healthcare is one of those activities.

Let's say you wake up one morning feeling ill. You explain to your AI-enhanced home platform that you are not feeling well. A series of sensors interact with you to determine if you have a fever, an elevated heart rate, or an abnormal respiratory rate. Trained to recognize your voice, your AI-enhanced platform detects a slight distortion. Based on the data, it calls a telehealth connection to schedule a virtual visit with your provider to confirm symptoms. With the help of additional AI-enhanced diagnostic tests (e.g., a rapid strep test), the nurse practitioner does an assessment that comes up with a diagnosis of streptococcus infection.

Your provider then arranges for the appropriate antibiotic treatment to be delivered. Because all your drug allergies and established medical history are stored on the AI-enhanced EHR, you do not need to worry about incorrect dosages, allergic reactions, or drug interactions when you take your prescription. With more help from AI, your provider shares a professional, compassionate, and comprehensive care plan, and continues to assess if your treatment is succeeding. Although this scenario is fictitious, the AI technologies to make it reality already exist.

AI is fundamentally transforming the relationship among patients, providers, and machines. This trend will only continue in the coming years and will be more pronounced in Millennials and younger generations.

Like electricity has become the general-purpose technology of our era, so will AI further the goals of medicine in the very near future. Healthcare strategies are already leveraging AI to create better, stronger, and more relevant medical tools to support our communities' health and resilience. AI will improve healthcare delivery value, reduce healthcare costs, promote accountability and collaboration among providers while improving the healthcare delivery infrastructure.

The AI revolution is not coming. It's already here.

AI Changing Lives

A Purpose for AI: Early Cancer Detection

The DoD JAIC is saving costs and lives with Google's prototype augmented reality microscope, which reduces the time it takes to review biopsies for breast and prostate cancers. The microscope uses a beam splitter to copy the image and pass it on to a high-resolution, high-speed digital camera. The camera instantly relays those images to the pathologist for analysis.

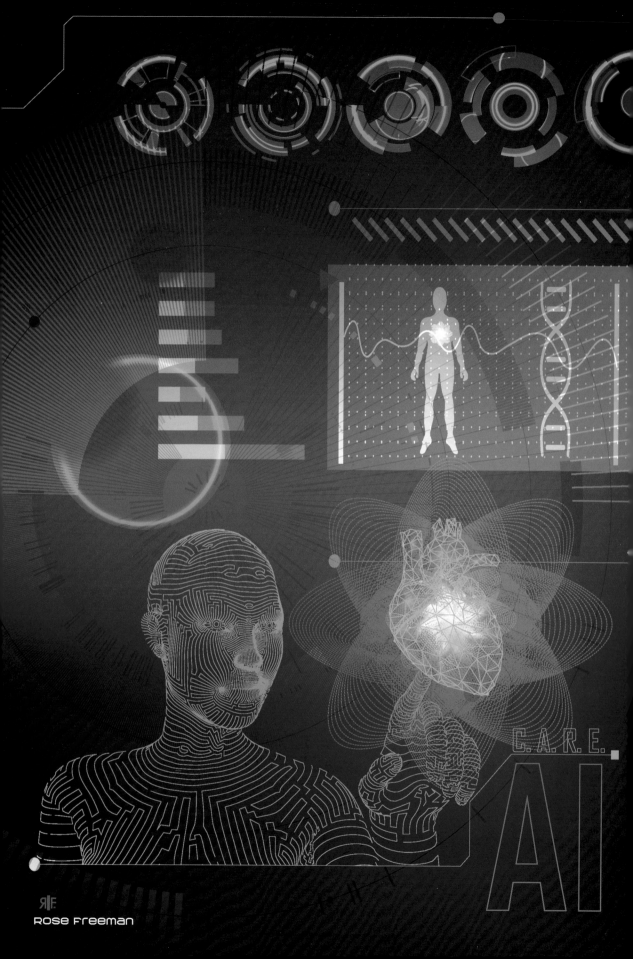

C.A.R.E.
AI

ROSE FREEMAN

C.A.R.E.

Adopting an AI-enhanced C.A.R.E. model strategy has great potential to enrich analytical systems, contain costs, and improve healthcare quality and outcomes.

C. Collect clinical data.

A. Analyze collected clinical data.

R. Risk-adjust clinical outcomes and data reporting.

E. Evaluate providers, group practice, and performance through feedback and practice outcome comparisons.

The C.A.R.E. model improves healthcare delivery system value, refocuses incentives for quality and reduces healthcare costs, promotes healthcare program accountability and collaboration, improves healthcare delivery infrastructure, and strengthens the provider's role through better data administration and establishing health care standards.

If you can't measure something, you can't improve it. An AI-enhanced data collection and evaluation process not only strengthens objective assessment but also improves healthcare delivery by predicting where a patient's health is heading while providing preventive solutions to maintain optimal wellness.

THE ART OF HUMAN CARE
IN ACTION

Still Chasing Nirvana with AI

*In 2010, a younger Dr. Tetteh wrote an audacious article,
"Achieving Nirvana through an Electronic Medical Record System:
A Military Surgeon's Perspective."[1] The intent was to share a vision
of an ideal condition of harmony, stability, and joy emanating from
an electronic medical record (EMR). I espoused my work from 1996
with the Veterans Health Information Systems and Technology
Architecture (VISTA) from the Veterans Affairs (VA). I highlighted
my experience with pilot modernization efforts with the Department
of Defense's (DoD) Armed Forces Health Longitudinal Technology
Application (AHLTA). Most importantly, I shared how we could
achieve EMR nirvana by adopting a framework advanced by
Howard Gardner in his book* Five Minds for the Future. *In his*

1 Tetteh, H. A. (2010). Achieving nirvana through an electronic medical record system: A military surgeon's perspective. *Military Medicine, 175*(5), 295–297. doi:10.7205/milmed-d-09-00102

work, Gardner identified five capacities or "minds" that we need to develop in order to be successful in the future.

From my perspective, each mind was ascribed to a platform. I outlined how a (1) disciplined (2) synthesizing, (3) creating, (4) respectful, and (5) ethical mind could work in concert to achieve EMR Nirvana. In 2010, the future end-state I envisioned was an electronic health record or EMR that would brilliantly serve healthcare providers with the ability to inform their clinical practice, interconnect providers, personalize care, and improve population health. Indeed, a decade ago, the goals were lofty. Many would argue that the goals still seem elusive today, yet progress has been made.

In my perspective, I also offered that true nirvana could be achieved if someday the Department of Defense's AHLTA system had interoperability with the Veterans Affairs VISTA system. In 2010, to mention such a paradigm was akin to blasphemy. Individuals tried for years to bring this idea to fruition without much success. In recent years, new investments in the commercial off-the-shelf Cerner solution now promise to replace the legacy AHLTA and VISTA systems and potentially unify a service member's electronic health record from enlistment through retirement. Furthermore, with interoperability standards advanced through policy and regulatory channels, there is potential for an electronic health record to exist on an individual from the time of birth to death. A so-called from-lust-to-dust archive of a human's entire health record can now exist in electronic format. Again, progress has been made.

The brilliance of a framework is that it allows complex material to be easily understood. When frameworks are excellent, like Gardner's, they endure the test of time and have evergreen utility. To that end, I am still chasing nirvana and believe AI nirvana can be achieved as the five disciplined, synthesizing, creating, respectful, and ethical capacities are applied to AI, as it represents an intelligent application.

A disciplined capacity inherently requires continual improvement beyond the initial acquisition of knowledge. AI applications will constantly evolve and need continual learning in order to cultivate perpetual improvement. Thus, AI applications in healthcare will require continual improvement based on new and evolving research and knowledge in order to provide the best insights and serve both healthcare providers and their patients.

We have moved well beyond the analog era. The burgeoning information age will continue to inundate the healthcare landscape. The challenge for healthcare providers will become more significant but AI applications may ease the burden if they can synthesize and filter what is most important and essential for patients. To help providers determine what matters most to patients in their personalized care will be crucial. Future AI applications' synthesizing capacity to analyze data, unify data from disparate sources, and furnish providers with relevant insight to assist and augment patient care will be paramount.

As an artist, I have long considered the definition of creativity. For me, creativity has always meant making connections. Whether the reference is made with a painter's brush to canvas, a sculptor's hand to spinning clay, a percussionist's beat to the drum, or the feeling one gets from hearing the song of poetry, creativity makes connections. In healthcare, a creating capacity in an AI application means an ability to connect the right solution with the right person at the right time. To have a high creating capacity is to make meaningful connections within the appropriate context for the problem or challenge at hand.

AI applications will serve more and more critical roles in healthcare as they mature and evolve. In the respectful capacity context, manipulations to algorithms and new machine learning initiatives must be made judiciously and always with empathy to the patients they will ultimately impact. AI applications should not be deployed in administrative vacuums without the sage and experienced contributions of informed healthcare providers and other stakeholders—including patients. In this way, we will consider and capture critical perspectives that ensure patient safety and guard against patient harm.

AI solutions and applications' ethical capacity will be advanced if providers, administrators, developers, and stakeholders define themselves within a community dedicated to caring for other humans. More than a decade ago, I evoked the concept of the **summum bonum,** *supreme good. In the ethical capacity of AI, reflection on the supreme good is appropriate and necessary. As we advance AI and chase nirvana for tomorrow, we must keep in mind that our goal is to improve patients' care. Indeed, we are all one heartbeat away from being a patient ourselves, our lives in the hands of the AI systems we ultimately create.*

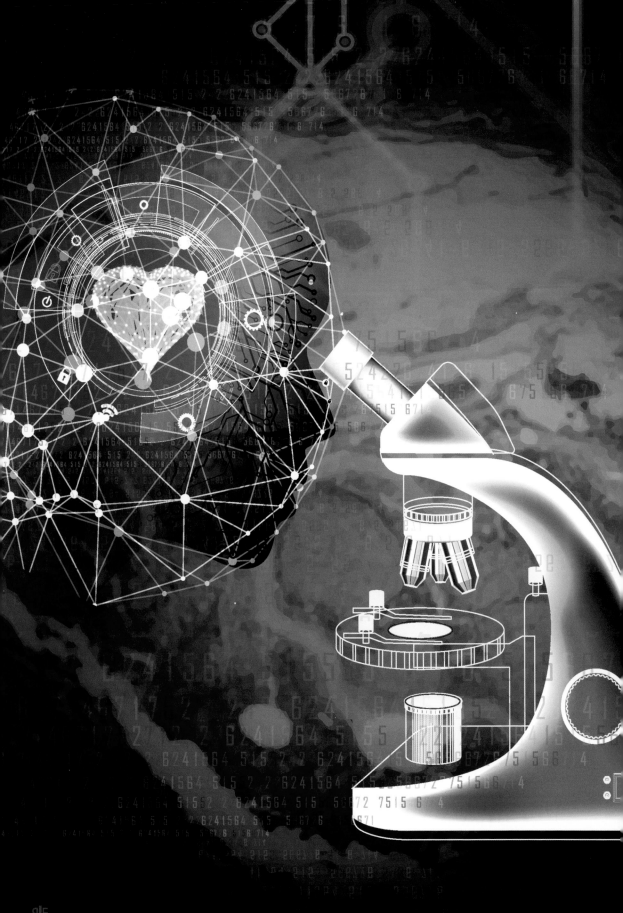

CHAPTER 3

ENHANCE
YOUR PURPOSE

I absolutely love what I do. Can I say that again? I love what I do. I love doing transplants. And I loved my role as Chief Medical Informatics Officer with the United States Navy. I'm excited about what AI can do for healthcare. My purpose in this chapter is to get you excited about it, too—and to explore some of the amazing opportunities that are before us.

I grew up in a little town in New York called Brooklyn. That was well over 25 years ago, and it was a different kind of Brooklyn. I dreamed of becoming a doctor. After completing my undergrad in a little arts and science college upstate New York, I received word that I had been selected for an interview at Johns Hopkins. But before the interview took place, I almost died of bacterial meningitis. That experience amplified my purpose in life, to be a physician. It also gave me perspective on what it feels like to be a patient. Ultimately, Johns Hopkins rejected me, but I still became a doctor. Over the course of my career, I developed my *Theory of Human Care*.

I've applied my philosophy to everything I do, whether I'm taking care of a patient in front of me, harvesting an organ for transplant, or working for the JAIC.

What is human care? It is delivering the kind of care you want delivered to you when you are in your most vulnerable position as a patient—when they take away your clothes and put you in one of those unflattering gowns, and when you're told you have something that could actually kill you or they inform you of some grave disease you've never heard of.

When you are in that place of vulnerability, you want someone to really care about you. You want someone to have compassion. That's what human care is. But it's more than that. It's delivering a comprehensive, holistic kind of care.

The three tenets of human care are purpose, personalization, and partnerships. Let's talk about your purpose. When you're gravely ill, what really motivates your recovery is your purpose—your will to be alive, to see your family, to see your grandkids, to accomplish more goals.

I love transplant. We have a purpose. We're trying to help someone who has a failed organ. In my discipline, it's a heart or lung that's no longer working and a patient who is going to die without that lifesaving, transplanted organ.

I've had an amazing career. I've gone all over the world. I've served as a ship's surgeon aboard the *USS Carl Vinson* (CVN 70) during Operation Iraqi Freedom. I've deployed as a trauma surgeon to Afghanistan during Operation Enduring Freedom. I've supported special joint forces missions to South America, the Middle East, the South Pacific, Australia, and Africa. Most recently, as I mentioned, I was recruited to lead an initiative at the JAIC, the Department of Defense's (DoD's) center of excellence for AI.

You may recall at the end of the George W. Bush administration and the beginning of the Obama administration, a full government AI strategy was espoused. All government entities were encouraged to develop an AI strategy that aligns with national security and AI advancement. The DoD's response was the JAIC. Established in 2018, its key objective is to deliver and advance AI capability and transform the DoD.

My health mission team's goal is to deliver AI-enabled capability across the military medicine enterprise. It's awesome and exciting work. It's a huge opportunity. But it's also a great challenge.

What's the first step to meeting any challenge? It's finding out why—discovering your purpose. The military has a strategic imperative to promote service members' health. We need healthy troops for mission success and to keep the nation secure. As a healer, my purpose is to support mission success for the warfighter and my patients. I want to help our service members who are ill, wounded, or injured to recover, get back to their service, and live full and happy lives. I want all my patients to do well. And I want my transplant patients to receive healthy organs in a timely manner in order to send them on the road of recovery to live full lives.

AI is already helping me achieve that purpose.

Finding Purpose
in War's Desert

When I landed in Afghanistan, stepping into the Helmand Province 120-degree heat was disorienting. But the needs of so many injured soldiers motivated me to work quickly.

By comparison, performing surgery in a hospital stateside is tame. The operating room is sterile. We work at a reasonable pace. We have the luxury of time to close the wounds delicately so friends and loved ones hardly notice the scar.

On the front line, surgery is down and dirty. We treated a gauntlet of men, and sometimes women, working as quickly as possible to save their lives after an explosion or enemy fire had blown them onto death's doorstep.

At first, the other surgeons and I felt dispirited. In addition to facing constant carnage, the conditions in our location were extremely austere. We had only the bare essentials necessary to save lives.

We engineered creative ways to stay connected with family. We even acquired a satellite to provide our team with an Internet connection that allowed us to keep in touch with loved ones back home. The provision of that technology was consequential and served us well, easing some of the pain of separation and isolation. As our tour ended, we matured, and my fellow surgeons and I realized our desert assignment was superior to the posh conditions our peers had been working in.

We lived hard. We were closer to the injured than ever before. We helped a lot of young service members who had been literally ripped apart by war. We gave them a shot at a future through our teamwork, tenacity, and dedication. In our sliver of the Afghan desert, in sagging tents, we cared for and supported our brave warriors. But some days, we lost, and it was not enough.

I saw too much.

My inspiration came from pain—the pain that came from the challenges and destruction I faced in the desert. Because we had all volunteered to be there, a tremendous esprit de corps arose among us.

Caring for so many young people's wounds and lives forced me to revisit my purpose in life. When we stabilized lethally injured patients, rescuing them from death, we gave them more time to find and fulfill their own purpose. That was the gift of a second chance that we fought hard to give each patient in the operating room.

Through my own suffering as a witness to trauma and destruction emerged a wisdom that engendered me with great humility, promoted a deep sense of gratitude for surviving the experience, and expanded my capacity to love all the facets of my life even more.

AI Changing Lives

Personalizing AI: In a Heartbeat

Studies using AI to enhance electrocardiogram (ECG) results identified patients at increased risk for irregular heartbeat (a-fib) and death. One-third of the top 1 percent of predicted high-risk patients were diagnosed with a-fib within a year. Up until now, a stroke was often the first sign that a person had a-fib. AI prediction could be the first step to prevention for people prone to stroke and a-fib in the future.

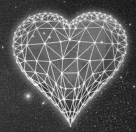

Part II

AI and personalization

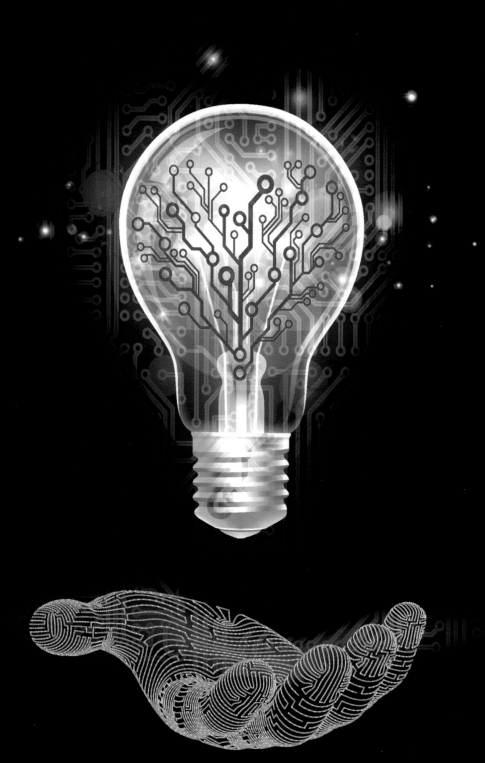

ROSE FREEMAN

chapter 4

HOW AI GOT
personal for me

What is going on in your world? No matter where you are in your world and who you are caring for, what is going on? When I take care of a patient, it's not enough for me to recognize that "something wrong" is going on with them, that something's happening, that a change is going on. Sometimes, it's hard to come up with a definitive answer as to what is going wrong.

Sometimes it's difficult to admit to yourself that you don't have the answer and that you may have to ask for help or go learn something new. It takes introspection and an understanding of your own personal situation to acknowledge that you don't have the skills to make that diagnosis.

Sometimes I have to get a second opinion. And I think, "Wouldn't it be great to get an instant second opinion from AI based on data that's seen exponentially more comparable cases than all of my colleagues and I have seen?"

Severence M. MacLaughlin, Ph.D., a colleague of mine at DeLorean Artificial Intelligence, believes that AI is going to provide what he calls "hyper-personalized care management." When you think DeLorean, maybe you think of the time-traveling car in the movie *Back to the Future*. In a sense, DeLorean AI is working on doing the same thing for the healthcare world. It is developing an AI system that can reference multiple data sources to make predictions about a patient's future—not just an analysis of the patient's past. DeLorean believes this AI system will give payers, providers, and patients better choices in care, better outcomes, less cost, and less hassle complying with all the regulatory paperwork.

Called Real Time Medical Care Management AI, this system of intelligence (SOI) develops mathematical profiles of patient journeys (symptoms, diagnoses, treatments) by sourcing information from insurance claims, pharmacy records, and data entered by their physicians, hospitals, and other sources. The AI is programmed to proactively intervene by selecting optimal treatments to prevent or address the progression of the specific diseases that the patient has or is predicted to develop. By predicting what the next best action patients and their care team should take, this AI has the goal of improving the patients' longevity and quality of care while reducing overall care management costs.

Now That's What I Call a Second Opinion!

Here's the thing about personalization. It requires an understanding of what's happening right now. And something is happening right now. Something big is happening. We are on the brink of a new era—a new dawn of AI, health, and creativity. And all it takes is for you to make it personal.

If you're doing human care really well, you personalize it to that specific person who is right in front of you. If you are a nurse, physician, or other healthcare provider, you personalize your healthcare to the patient you are with.

I've told countless medical students, residents, and even my own colleagues, "Have empathy." If there was a course in medical school, nursing school, and allied health where you could become a patient for a day, or even a few hours, it would be worth it.

Putting yourself in the shoes of the person you are taking care of on a day-to-day basis—every moment you engage with them— gives you a totally different experience. You don't only treat the heart if you are a heart surgeon. You don't only treat the brain if you are a neurologist. You don't only treat the toe if you are a podiatrist. Instead, you treat the whole person by taking a holistic approach. You do more than come up with a diagnosis and treatment plan. You practice personalized human care.

Think about the very special moments you've had when you were rendering care to a patient—the times you engaged with true empathy. Perhaps you were trying to make that person feel better. Or maybe you were trying to get them back to work or back to enjoying physical activity. You recognized that the therapies and treatments that work for one person may not be the approach suited for your patient. You personalized their care.

Make AI Personal for You

When I talk about personalization, I suggest you think about the innovations you can achieve with AI. Think about the dreams you've had to improve something in your work or discipline. My dream is to improve heart and lung transplantation, save more lives, and improve outcomes for patients. Through the work of our Specialized Transplant AI-Adaptive Recovery (STAR) Teams, we are applying analytics to the rich data we have collected over a decade and leveraging AI to gain invaluable insights that are already improving our work. Consider the gaps in terms of what you know now and what you need to learn. What skills need retooling? What knowledge is missing? How can we make things better with the general-purpose technology of our era?

This was a lesson for me, and it's a broader lesson for all of us. We can passively use the technology that's become part of our daily lives, or we can think beyond our laptops and smartphones to embrace new ways of using AI to enhance our personal experience, our professional experience, and the way we experience caring for each other.

AI Changing Lives

Personalizing AI: What's the Good Word?

A team from IBM and Pfizer are training AI models to screen for Alzheimer's disease by analyzing patterns in word usage. Other researchers are doing the same by employing AI to analyze brain scans and clinical test results. As a result, Alzheimer's could be predicted years before symptoms become severe enough for typical diagnosis—and word analysis is much less invasive than the current tests and scans. Early diagnosis means earlier treatment and better outcomes for Alzheimer's patients.

THE ART OF HUMAN CARE
IN ACTION

Teach
Your Parents Well

I was very comfortable as a general surgeon—and I liked cardiac surgery. I got good at it, but even so, there were times I needed to learn more. Then I discovered informatics. I didn't know a lot about it. I knew it involved computers. I knew it involved data. I decided I needed to know more. But here's the great thing: my son was the one who pointed me in the right direction.

Long before I heard about informatics, I gave my son the nickname Wisdom. Soon after he was born, we were visiting my mother-in-law. Her next-door neighbor, an older woman, saw us going into the house from the car with the cradle and the little car seat. The old woman looked like a person who had a lot of knowledge about life. She stopped me and said, "Your son is going to bring you great wisdom." I thought to myself, "What is this old lady talking about?"

If you've had children, and I'm sure many of you have, you know that they do bring you wisdom. Sometimes they say things that make you open your mind and heart to new possibilities.

This was one of those times, and one I'll never forget. I had just returned from one of my deployments when my son was about eight years old (he is now 16). My wife and I were driving. My daughter was in her car seat. My son was buckled up in the back seat. We were talking, for some reason, about college. Naturally, our kids were going to go to college, right? I mean, that was a no-brainer, not even a debate. We seared that into their heads from early on, no question. So we're driving, and my son says, "I'm not going to go to college."

His mother and I were like, "What? Stop the car. What's happening? Where did this come from? Who told you this?"

I turned around and said, "What are you talking about, Edmund? What do you mean, you're not going to college?" He said, "Dad, I can learn everything I need to know on YouTube."

Eight years ago, that seemed like nonsense to me. But right now, people are actually getting certificates in cooking, gardening, and all kinds of other things from YouTube. You want to learn how to change a carburetor in a 1967 Ford? Look it up on YouTube. Some dude or some woman will come on screen and say, "Let me tell you what you've got to do. You've got to turn this thing and turn that thing and get this tool."

When my eight-year-old son started talking about this thing called YouTube, I realized that we are in an age when there are all kinds of opportunities to learn online through Udemy, Coursera, and more.

I am a perpetual student. I love to go to school. I mean, I really love it. I'm just naturally curious. I remember when I was talking to an admissions advisor after being accepted into a master's program for AI, the first AI online course Johns Hopkins University offered through its engineering school.

As we talked, the admissions advisor asked, "What are you doing this for?"

I said, "Oh, I'm just interested. I think if I'm going to do the work, I should get some kind of credit for it. I want to get a certificate."

He said, "You know, I think you have enough degrees. You know what you should do? Just take a course in the subject that you want to learn about. That's all you need to do at this stage. You don't have to prove anything to anybody anymore."

I thought, "Not a bad idea."

My point is that you can learn any of this stuff, and it's virtually free.

Where did my son get his wisdom? It was his personalization of his own situation. At eight years old, he loved video games; he loves them even more now. But he couldn't finish a lot of the video games, and he couldn't pass certain levels. I would come downstairs and see him doing this very peculiar thing. He would be playing his game while he had a video playing. I heard people talking. I thought, "What is this kid doing? Why has he got all this stuff going on?" I found out that he was watching another player on YouTube who had mastered the game.

That's why he said in the car that day, "Dad, why do I have to go to college? I can learn everything I want on YouTube."

Now let me make this clear; he's still going to go to college. I'm proud to say he's in Georgetown Preparatory High School, getting ready for college. We've made a big investment in order to get that thought out of his head, that thought about settling for YouTube U. But on the other hand, my son, Wisdom, lived up to his nickname that day. He took what he learned from his own personal experience and expanded upon it. By interacting with the technology available to him—video games and Youtube—he found ways to succeed in his "practice," gaming.

AI Changing Lives

AI and MATH: SOMETHING NEW IS ON THE HORIZON

Will human mathematicians soon become obsolete? The first truly creative proof of a mathematical theorem by an artificial intelligence (AI) is on the horizon. We should be filled with both excitement and anxiety in equal measure.

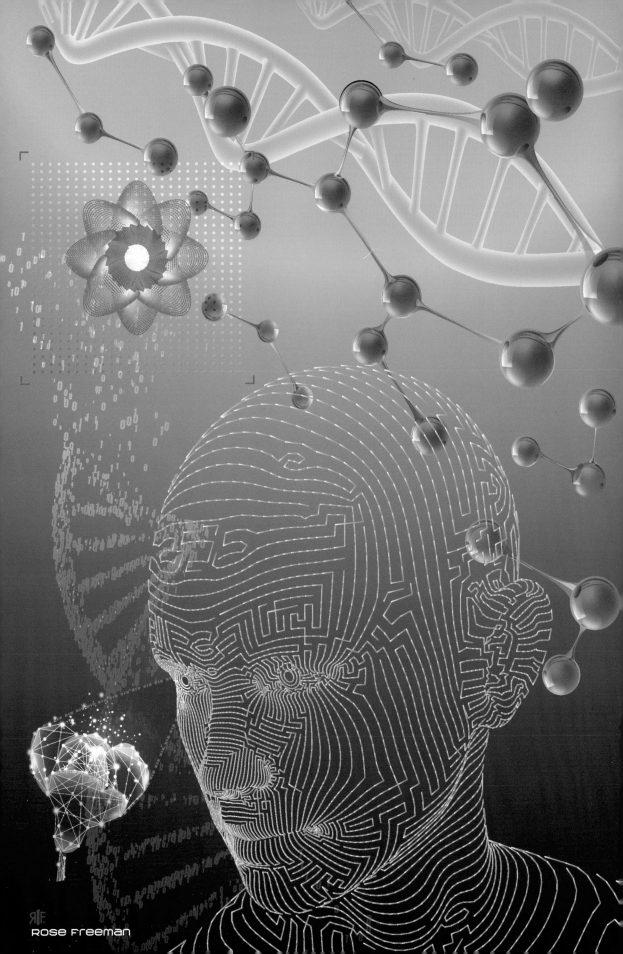
ROSE FREEMAN

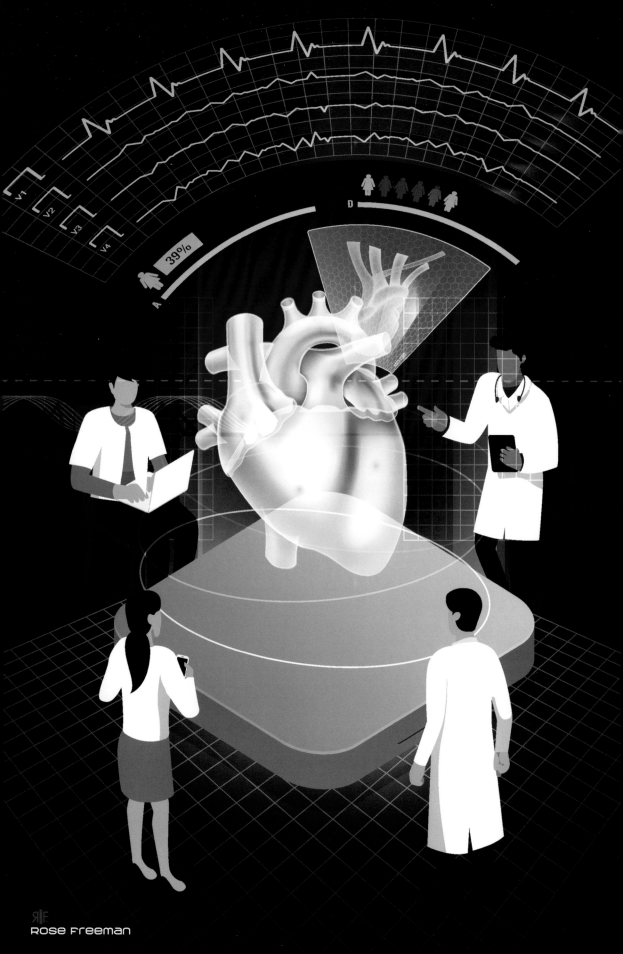

ROSE FREEMAN

Chapter 5

How AI Can Make It Personal For You

Despite the changes to healthcare legislation that were signed into law in 2010, issues of affordable cost, equitable access, and consistent quality have continued to dominate the current debate on healthcare in the United States. However, the new paradigm of AI-enhanced healthcare delivery addresses all three. In fact, some savvy healthcare providers are already using technology to solve these issues—and they're also discovering that AI helps them to better personalize that care.

For example, we all know what a tablet is today. We've even seen children playing games on them. A New York City orthodontist, Dr. Ferencz, was an early tablet adopter. He has employed the tablet to realize true cost and practice benefits. The tablet is now central to all aspects of his practice. It simplifies patient forms and record-keeping and enables him to show his patients photos of various treatment options. His technicians refer to digital images on the tablet to create perfect-looking prosthetics. With the tablet, Dr. Ferencz achieves a seamless transfer of data from doctor to patient to technician that improves efficiency, reduces the space needed for records, and saves costs and time. "With [the tablet], we save so much time—and space," he says.

This technology also enables Dr. Ferencz to personalize his care for his patients. The tablet shows patients exactly how particular prosthetics will be applied. And he uses the device to communicate more effectively with patients. Because patients have a visual idea of how the procedure takes place, they can anticipate their outcome. The result is a direct improvement in care. "[The tablet] is ideally suited to this kind of visual conversation," he says. "The patient and I can flip through the X-rays and clinical photos together, and I can illustrate my points as we go."

The tablet is one example of readily available technology that can immediately inform physicians of the cost of diagnostic tests and medications in real time, help inform care plan decisions with cost consciousness in mind, use email to communicate to patients, and share patient data with other health care providers for more efficient patient care coordination.

Personalizing care is one benefit of AI-enhanced healthcare. Other benefits I believe we will see include informing clinical practice, interconnecting providers, and improving population health. However, personalizing care may be the most important benefit. When people think about AI and healthcare, they might imagine cold robotic nurses, stark walls of machines, and care taking place in sterile isolation.

Just the opposite is true. In an ever-advancing science that has become more and more reliant on computers and technology, medicine can utilize AI to create the tools providers need in order to get to know their patients better—and increase the amount of time they have to spend face-to-face with them. AI might just be the thing to get physicians' eyes off their laptop screens and back on their patients. AI can make the space for "heart" to fully come back into the practice of medicine.

A Heartfelt, Deeply Personal Practice of Medicine

Life is full of twists and turns. Every experience you have is a lesson on your never-ending journey of personal discovery. Living each day heartfelt and engaged is the best way to ensure the purpose of each experience and lesson is discovered. Such discovery is often elusive. Lessons learned from disappointment are not immediately obvious, especially in our impatient, modern society. Take time to pause and see the beauty of your daily experiences—both the highs and the lows.

If you want to live from the heart, you cannot afford to give up trying. You must never give up trying to achieve your goals and dreams. Do not allow days and weeks to go by without personal reflection. It's natural to focus on what you haven't done today, last month, or this year. Instead, focus on what you have done and accomplished. You will find peace and strength. Never give up! Your continued effort, despite the challenges, is what will accomplish your goals.

On August 3, 1857, Frederick Douglass delivered a "West India Emancipation" speech in Canandaigua, New York. Most of his address centered on the history of British emancipation efforts as well as a reminder of the vital role that West Indian slaves played in the struggle for freedom. Douglass spoke presciently of the coming Civil War and at the tail end of his speech produced one of the most quoted sentences of all his public speeches: "If there is no struggle, there is no progress." This simple sentence underscores the importance of persistence and the relentless pursuit of heartfelt living.

You can never afford to give up on your goals, objectives, and dreams. As long as you are still alive, each day offers a new opportunity to progress, accomplish your goals, and become great. When you focus on the important things, your life has purpose and meaning, and you will feel alive. As you pursue your own personal goals, be sure to do the following:

- Maintain your health. You have one body, one life, one chance here on earth to live. Honor yourself by taking care of your mind, body, and spirit daily.

- Do work you enjoy. Organized action, which you are compensated for, requires a strong work ethic, consistency, and discipline, and will bring reward when you enjoy what you do.

- Give and receive love. Without love the world can be a cold place. We are social and need to love and receive love. Look around for love, whether it is from family members, lovers, friends, and acquaintances, or just in the eyes of loving people you connect with. The perceivable presence of love is vital.

- Maintain a peaceful environment. Take command of your environment, and make an effort to establish peace at all times.

- Keep good friends, and be a good friend. Fight to keep loyal, giving, understanding friends in your life who want nothing from you but your friendship in return.

- Grow through change. If you feel as if you've "arrived," that is an invitation to learn something new about yourself and the life you've been given. Take on a new challenge! Change is inevitable, so embrace it and prepare for the personal growth it brings. Embrace the change with your whole heart.

For the older generations, AI technology is one of the twists and turns we were not expecting to impact the way we did our jobs. But whether we are ready or not, technology is changing the parameters of medicine. We also may not have expected to be spending so much of our time dealing with forms, red tape, compliance, and data. AI can relieve that. AI-enhanced medicine does not look like the cold, impersonal portrayals of dystopian futures that we see at the movies. It looks a lot more personal. AI can help us untangle the codes, costs, and confusion caused by mountains of untethered data and paperwork requirements and make more room for conversation, caring, and the personalization that helps us all feel a little more human. AI-enhanced medicine can make more room for the heart.

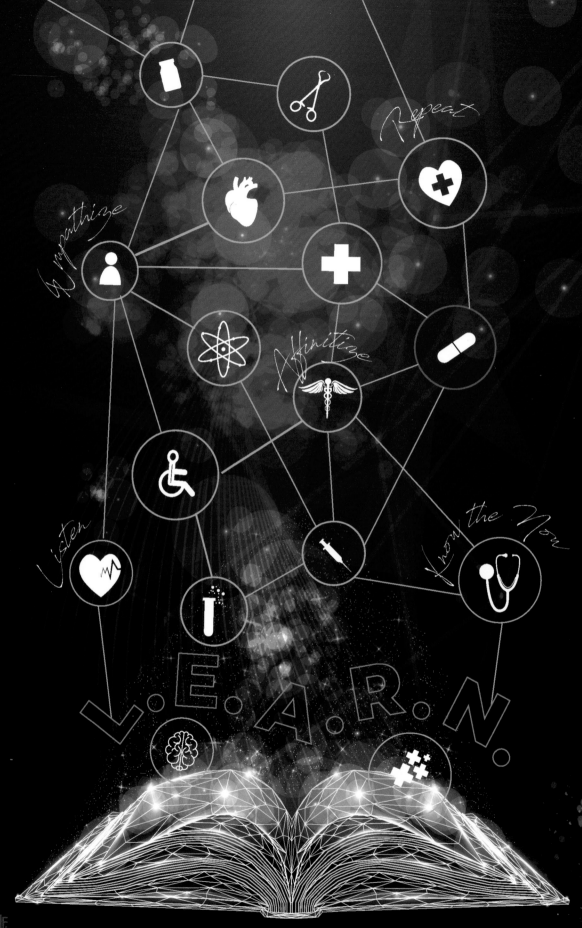

L.E.A.R.N.

No matter how far AI takes us into the future of medicine, the importance of personalizing our relationships with those we treat, serve, or care for will never become obsolete. The acronym L.E.A.R.N. can guide you in personalizing your work and relationships.

L. Listen

In my first year of medical school at SUNY Downstate Medical Center, Dr. Friedman admonished that if we listen to the patient, truly listen to the patient, "They will tell you the diagnosis." This has proved true every time I've truly listened to my patient. If you want to change the world, you must listen to your clients, patients, friends, and family—really listen to them.

E. Empathize

My deathbed experience as a patient in the ICU taught me about empathy. I know what it feels like to be a patient. If, as a healthcare provider or family caregiver, you want to change the world, you must empathize with the people in your life and what they are experiencing. You must imagine walking in their shoes. That will help you better understand their pain and situation.

A. Affinitize

Even more important, learn to affinitize with clients, patients, friends, and family before telling them what they need to do. What matters most to them—their job, hobbies, family activities, volunteer work? If you want to change the world, you must affinitize with the people you serve before prescribing them a plan of action. Make sure your advice or treatment addresses what matters most to them.

R. Repeat

When people need help, they most likely are under a great deal of stress. It may take some reinforcement to really drive a point home. Repetition is important. If you want to change the world, you must repeat important messages to the person you are caring for and again to their family members. Make sure lines of communication are clear and that you answer all questions and concerns.

N. Know the Now

Know what the person's greatest current concern is—right now, today. For example, a patient, client, or loved one with diabetes may not care about HgbA1C. But they might do whatever it takes to love and care for their children or grandchildren—now and in the future. If you want to change the world, know what the person's concern is now. Remember, the answer will only come from the person you are caring for.

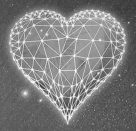

Part III

AI and Partnerships

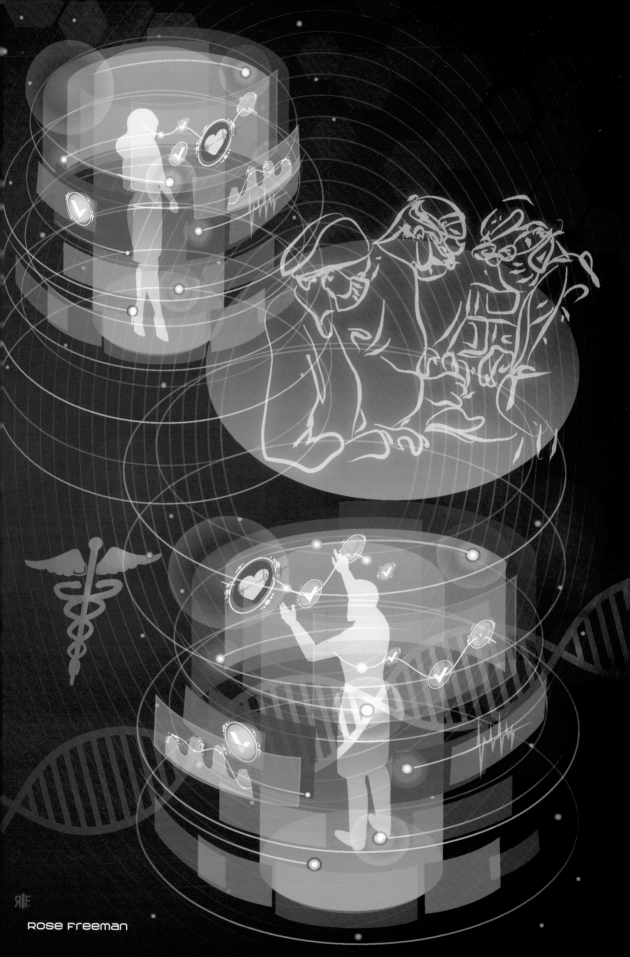

ROSE FREEMAN

Chapter 6

Human Partnerships Determine AI Success

How do we do it? How do we deliver AI-enabled capability? I can tell you that it's a learning process. Many of you are doing it right now in your respective domains. I can also tell you that after studying AI for many years—and even in my last role as U.S. Navy chief medical informatics officer—every day I learn something new.

That's because AI is a brand-new space. It's a blank canvas. The textbook to tell you how to do it hasn't been written yet. And maybe it never will be because the AI of today is not going to be the AI of tomorrow. That makes AI even more challenging but also even more exciting. However, I believe that by following a framework of purpose, personalization, and partnerships, we will achieve great goals using AI in healthcare. Developing the right partnerships will make the impossible possible. I have learned so much from the folks I've engaged with because there is so much information to be learned from those who are doing this work. And partnerships are a great way to make that happen.

In the previous chapters, we talked about purpose. And we talked about personalization. Now let's talk about partnerships. AI cannot be developed in a vacuum. We will not succeed in our purpose if we develop solutions and then go out to find problems. What we need to do is engage with our stakeholders across the medical community, understand their problems, and then pursue the AI-enabled capabilities that solve those problems. With that iterative process, I've seen incredible things happen.

There are developments on the AI horizon that many of my clinical colleagues don't even know about. Through engagements with AI innovators, we have learned of AI solutions with great potential utility in healthcare. For example, we have an incredible amount of information on our service members. If you think about it, we begin collecting health information from recruits as soon as they sign on. They may be as young as seventeen years old. Throughout their military career, we continue to collect health data, whether they remain enlisted for four years, fourteen years, or forty. When they retire or are discharged, we continue collecting their data as we provide care for them through Veterans Affairs (VA).

We have comprehensive data on millions of individuals. Notably, we have over 100 million digitized radiographic studies and more than 55 million pathology slides that have been collected over the course of a century and not yet digitized. Collectively, this is a rich data resource and significant machine learning opportunity.

One of our goals is to accelerate health classification so we can do better diagnoses. How do we do that? We evolve partnerships with public entities, private industry, academia, the cyber community, and anyone else that has a novel idea that could help develop the solution. AI innovation requires continuous and evolving learning, communication with leaders in the field, and appreciating what others are working on.

By having these kinds of conversations and these types of engagements, we can learn from each other and realize, "Hey, we have a problem. There's a solution or a potential solution. We can work together."

Military medicine applies to a lot of areas in the civilian sector as well. You cannot deploy, sustain, and scale AI unless you have a massive amount of infrastructure. One conclusion I made is that this is an exciting place to be right now.

The DoD is the expert in dealing with data. It has the computer power, the storage power, the expertise, the engineers, and the computer scientists. It deals with a wealth of data. This gives us a foundation, an infrastructure. With the data, the tools, the storage, and the computing power that enable us to develop the algorithms, we can do the machine learning that's necessary.

From a machine learning algorithm standpoint, we curate the data and condition it. One of my AI colleagues at the VA says we're making data "AI-able." That is not an easy thing to do at times, especially for healthcare, but that's what we're doing.

By training the algorithms, doing the testing, and making the evaluations, we can deliver capabilities in the areas I mentioned before. Health records analysis is like finding that golden needle in the haystack. It involves sifting through all the information in order to get the necessary insight. When it comes to medical imaging, petabytes of radiographic as well as pathology imaging exists. And we are using computer vision to advance, develop, and help with diagnostic capabilities.

Automated medical logistics help us deliver care to very austere places. That will help us better treat patients at their point of injury, even when our campaigns—particularly in the future—are in locations where we do not have the air superiority we enjoyed in the past. How do we deliver care and keep people alive when care may not be able to get to them for some time? Those are the problems we're working on.

There are new ways to think about the days ahead. Five things are driving this new agenda in AI.

- A massive amount of data.
- Incredible computing power.
- The electronic health record.
- Professionals that have developed machine learning algorithms that are way better than they were in the past.
- Government and commercial investments.

Thus, we have a convergence that makes this time a lot different. Even though AI's claims and fame have been rehashed for decades, I would argue that because my teenage son and my daughter keep staring at their smartphones, this time it's different.

Right now, we're engaging with academia, the commercial sector, and international partners. We know that this is such a new place, a new dawn, that not everyone has it right yet. We're learning from each other, and we are on the verge of forming partnerships with AI and each other that will truly revolutionize the practice of medicine.

THE ART OF HUMAN CARE
IN ACTION

seize
The moment

Consider this scenario. Mrs. Carter gets up from her couch and stumbles to the floor with sudden paralysis. Her husband recognizes the symptoms of stroke, realizes the emergency, and knows that time is critical. He foregoes calling 911 and takes her immediately to their nearby rural hospital. The small hospital does not have a neurologist on staff. However, they have telehealth technology and access to stroke neurologists and specialists at an urban hospital 70 miles away. A world-renowned neurologist is on call. He uses the video-conferencing link and web-based software to remotely assess the nature and severity of Mrs. Carter's stroke. After a careful and comprehensive review of tests, available information, patient history, and examination, the neurologist recommends the patient receive a clot-busting thrombolytic drug that is highly *effective when given in a timely manner for some stroke victims but can cause adverse events when given to others. Mrs. Carter is seen and treated within three hours of her stroke onset thanks to the quick response of her husband and rural hospital staff. Without the partnerships that telehealth made possible, she may have died. Instead, she makes a full recovery.*

Telehealth: The Next Frontier

Telehealth benefits the patient through improved healthcare outcomes as a result of timelier access to a specialist who can help deliver the highest standard of care to a patient in need. But in the above scenario, Mrs. Carter is not the only beneficiary. Consider the rural hospital where she received care. By utilizing telehealth care, the hospital retains the patient, and she can remain close to home with her husband and family. Still the benefits continue. The neurologist who provides the care remotely is able to extend clinical reach to patients who benefit from his or her expertise.

Telehealth care is rapidly becoming conventional for healthcare organizations around the globe. More than 2,000 telehealth studies have demonstrated the value of remote healthcare. Results include reduced hospital readmissions, decreased home nursing visits, and lower overall costs. Additionally, patients and caregivers who use telehealth technologies have reported increased satisfaction with treatments. These findings have encouraged many countries to integrate more remote healthcare into their current healthcare practices.

Medicine and Technology: A Long History

All generations of healthcare providers in modern history have partnered with advancing technology to improve and expand patient access to healthcare. Advancing technology turned ambulances into helicopters to provide swifter emergency care. New communications technology evolved clunky pen and paper memos and reports that could reach only a handful of folks into web-based correspondence that is easy to access, share globally, and store with just a few clicks.

As the COVID-19 pandemic demonstrated, technology has once again asserted momentum into healthcare access. Through the undeniable benefits of telehealth, millions of lives have been saved. Countless more patients can look forward to improved healthcare outcomes as the technology matures. The benefits are multiplying exponentially as more healthcare providers implement telehealth into their routine delivery of care. When physicians, healthcare systems, individual facilities, and patients partner via telehealth, everyone benefits.

The American Telemedicine Association says that telemedicine is the use of medical information exchanged from one site to another via electronic communications to improve patients' health statuses. However, the term telehealth *is used to encompass a broader definition of remote healthcare that does not always involve clinical services—but always involves partnership.*

Videoconferencing, transmission of still images, e-health including patient portals, remote monitoring of vital signs, continuing medical education, and nursing call centers are all considered part of telemedicine and telehealth.

Although some debate over telehealth's efficacy continues, clearly defining telehealth is necessary. The Health Resources Services Administration defines it as "the use of electronic information and telecommunications technologies to support long-distance clinical healthcare, patient and professional health-related education, public health and health administration." Videoconferencing, the internet, store-and-forward imaging, streaming media, and terrestrial and wireless communications support a wealth of platforms.

The use of telehealth to facilitate partnerships in healthcare will continue to grow in the United States as technology matures and the nature of our healthcare delivery evolves.

Partnerships:
AI Takes Aim at A1C

Precision Nutrition is helping people living with type 2 diabetes control their disease. The program partners AI and genomic analysis with registered dietitians, a personalized nutrition app, and healthcare providers to precisely develop diets that control patients' individual blood sugar levels. Patients mail a stool sample to DayTwo, the company that developed the program, to analyze the unique population of microbes found in their digestive systems.

By referencing a scoring system that rates thousands of foods and food combinations based on the individual's unique microbiome sample and DNA sequencing, the clinicians apply an algorithm to predict the foods that will cause blood sugar to spike. By referencing a linked phone app, patients can predict their glycemic response to specific foods and food combinations. Patients participating in a 2020 Saginaw, Michigan, pilot of the project reported having more energy, better sleep, less hunger, and reduced stress. Over the course of the three-month pilot, their A1C tests (a measure of average blood sugar) dropped an average of 1.6 points, and they lost an average of 18 pounds.

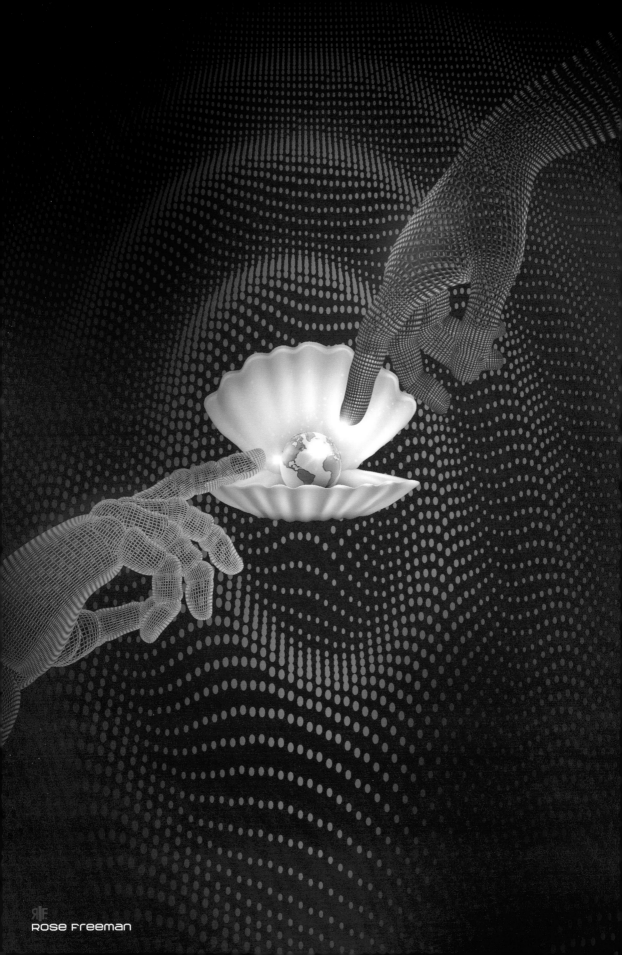

ROSE FREEMAN

Chapter 7

Engineer the Human into Everything You Do

When I was deployed as a surgeon to Afghanistan, tending to soldiers who had suffered terrible trauma and had been blown up by Improvised Explosive Devices (IEDs), it all came down to partnership with the other physicians, nurses, and medical staff. It meant partnership with the corpsmen and medevac teams and partnerships with the people who cleaned the surgery tents after we finished. We all knew we had a common purpose: to save these soldiers' lives and send them home to their families. Because of that partnership, we achieved amazing things—impossible things—in the middle of the desert.

Our partnerships worked because they were supported by three elements: caring, communicating, and creating a team around a shared vision and a mission. These are the only three things you need to know about building great partnerships. I repeat: caring, communicating, and creating a team.

If you're able to do those three things in your partnerships—personally, professionally, and organizationally—you can be a catalyst that changes the world.

The tent in Afghanistan where we operated doesn't exist anymore. That base where we were has all gone back to desert. But in that sliver of time, in that patch of sand, we did amazing things. We didn't have an MRI machine. We weren't even connected to gas, electric, or water lines. But we didn't need those things. We just needed to care. And we did. We absolutely cared about those soldiers who we were taking care of. We had the kind of caring that understood the human condition and wanted to help.

Just as important, we effectively communicated. It was always a challenge, as you can imagine, but we made a point of making true communication happen. No excuses. No "I didn't see your text" or "Your email got lost in the string" because communicating meant life, and failing to communicate meant death.

When you communicate effectively, you bring people together around a common goal. You craft your message, your vision and mission, the right way and create your team.

Because we cared and because we communicated, we created a great team with a shared vision. That vision kept us going when we were physically tired and emotionally empty. Because we were all aligned around a common mission, we did great things.

If you're able to create a common mission, establish good and open communication, and rally a bunch of people who care, anything is possible—especially today when AI can help us fill in the gaps. Mainstream healthcare professionals have many great resources available, amazing amenities, and fantastic hospitals. We have a great, talented cadre of people at our disposal to create awesome and amazing teams. We have no excuse to not make the impossible possible.

Partnerships Make It Happen

When a person tragically becomes an organ donor due to trauma or some unfortunate mishap, there's another person, or perhaps two or three, on the other end who will receive a great gift, the miracle of life itself. When my Specialized Thoracic Adapted Recovery (STAR) Team gets involved, it means we will be bringing somebody a new heart today. It's a good thing.

Transplant surgery is very exciting. It's one of those professions where you deal with life and death every day, every case. A life-saving organ! It's exhilarating. It's stressful. And at times it's unlike any other experience you could ever have in healthcare. It's an incredibly gratifying feeling to know we've brought this gift of life to another human being. We can play a small part in this group of people who are partnering to make this happen—the physicians, nurses, doctors, and coordinators.

It's not one person. It's not one team. It's a partnership that brings many teams together—the STAR team is just one of them. There are also teams from different hospitals, different specialties, different professions—doctors, nurses, transport, social workers, payors, clergy, even the cleaning crew. Yes, it feels sort of like being deployed to do surgery in Afghanistan—but without the desert. And now we have the opportunity to include a new partner that can bring an awful lot to the table: AI.

In the spring of 2019, my colleagues at the University of Maryland made the news when they delivered a kidney using an autonomous drone. They successfully demonstrated how AI can deliver transplant organs faster, more safely, and with fewer logistical problems like traffic jams than my STAR team driving across a few states in the middle of the night.

The innovation of this flight took partnerships among aviation and engineering experts at the University of Maryland's Department of Aerospace Engineering and Unmanned Aircraft Systems Test Site, the FAA, transplant physicians and researchers at the University of Maryland School of Medicine, and collaborators at the Living Legacy Foundation of Maryland.

This AI miracle brought a new kidney to a 44-year-old Baltimore resident who had spent eight long years on dialysis. This is why I love AI. And this is why I love transplant. Both are the embodiment of complete teamwork. Most importantly, partnerships are the only way it's possible to make human care successful—partnerships between the healthcare provider, the patient, the community, the government, and so many more people.

If you carry purpose, personalization, and partnerships in your heart, you will deliver compassionate, effective human care just like that drone delivered the kidney. You cannot even imagine the impact you will have on people's lives.

Engineer the human into everything you do; never engineer the human out. And when you see somebody or one of your colleagues engineering the human out, stop them. Be a vanguard. You have no excuse to not make the impossible possible.

THE ART OF HUMAN CARE
IN ACTION

Heroes
Never Stand Alone

The U.S. Military Health System does an outstanding job assisting our heroes during recovery. One component of the U.S. Military Health System, the Defense and Veterans Brain Injury Center, works tirelessly to serve active-duty military, their beneficiaries, and veterans with traumatic brain injuries.

Headquartered in the nation's capital, the DVBIC provides state-of-the-art clinical care, innovative research, and educational programs at sixteen sites. The Center's effectiveness has led the Department of Defense to name it the Office of Responsibility and charge it with additional tasks ranging from pre-deployment testing, managing data, and overseeing studies of service members with traumatic brain injuries to creating a family caregiver curriculum.

The DVBIC shares countless success stories. One of the most touching is Staff Sergeant Ben Ricard's road to recovery, as told by U.S. Department of Veterans Affairs.

In November 2009, Ricard was driving a Mine Resistant Ambush Protected vehicle when he hit a roadside improvised explosive device (IED). The blast blew him through the door of the vehicle. He broke his back, both of his legs, an arm, and suffered a traumatic brain injury. Following initial treatment at Langstuhl, Germany, and then Walter Reed Army Hospital, Ricard entered the Richmond Veteran's Affairs Polytrauma Rehabilitation Center to begin the recovery process.

After significant therapy and treatment, including learning to walk again, Ricard returned to an active-duty Marine Corps unit. Throughout his treatment and recovery, Ricard found strength in many sources: his wife, his children, his parents, his military training, and his belief in himself.

"I gradually got stronger," he said. "I was able to stand up. I was able to walk. I was able to hug my wife. I was able to hold my kids. No matter how tough it is, it gets better. That's the toughest thing to deal with because it takes time and it takes patience."

Another veteran, Charles Hargrove, served in the US military for 20 years. Returning from three tours of duty in 2007, he battled severe post-traumatic stress disorder (PTSD). Soon after returning home, he was fortunate enough to purchase his first home. Within a few days of becoming a homeowner, Hargrove found himself standing before a tornado-battered residence. With the help of the community and admirable inner strength, he rebuilt his home, only for it to burn to the ground seven months later.

In the midst of seemingly insurmountable turmoil, Hargrove decided to launch a non-profit organization, Wounded Warriors One Voice. His ultimate goal is to bring clothing and affordable wheelchairs throughout the country and restore the dignity of wounded warriors. Hargrove used his misfortune as motivation to do good in the world and serve others.

While these two heroes are shining examples of inner strength and perseverance, they also underscore the importance of reaching out in partnership. During their recoveries, they both joined in wholeheartedly as partners with their medical teams, family, and community. As a result, they made their own lives and their own communities a better place to live.

AI Changing Lives

Partnerships: Can AI End Animal Testing?

Instead of relying on mice, monkeys, cats, or dogs, pharmaceutical companies may soon be using AI-enhanced "organs-on-chips" to simulate human organs as they work on developing new drugs. These will not only save thousands of animals from suffering and death, but also decrease pharmaceutical development costs.

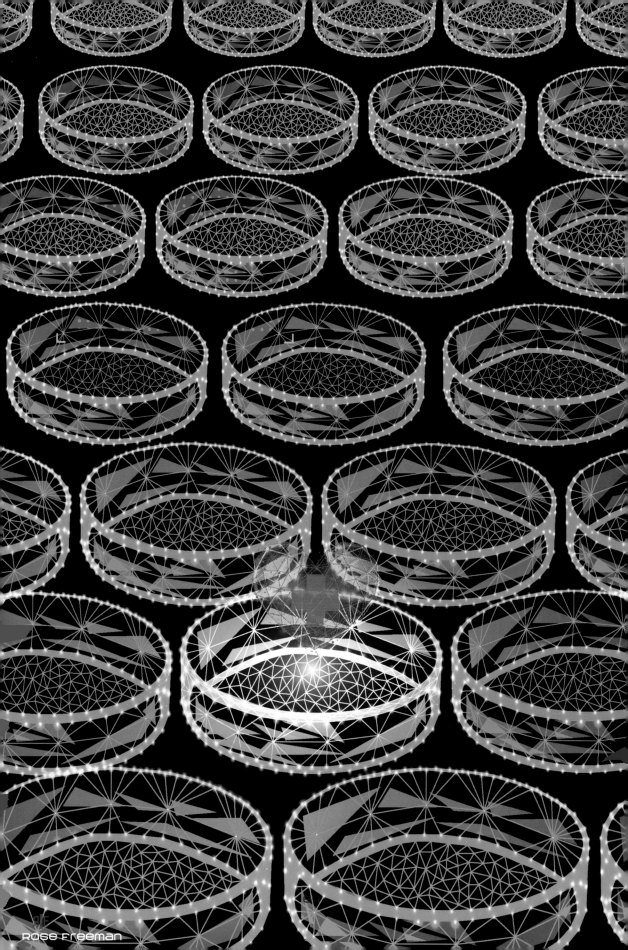

Chapter 8

The Future
is Now

AI is in the news. According to a recent *Forbes* article, doctors using a new AI-driven neural network can detect heart failure from a single heartbeat with 100 percent accuracy. *CDO Trends* reported that 69 percent of what managers currently do will be automated in the coming years. The COVID-19 pandemic accelerated the adoption of AI and industrial automation, according to *Analytics India Magazine*.

In February of 2021, my colleagues at the Department of Defense Joint Artificial Intelligence Center (DoD JAIC) published an interesting online article, "The Right Information in the Right Hands at the Right Time," about its MERIT project. MERIT stands for Medical Evaluation Readiness Information Tools. It shares how MERIT uses AI capabilities to predict service members' health status. Currently, MERIT focuses on seven conditions common among service members—asthma, arthritis, limited motion in arm and leg, residuals of traumatic brain injury, intervertebral disc syndrome, and major depression—and expects to expand that to twenty conditions that 90 percent of service members with disabilities commonly have. While MERIT does not make any clinical decisions, it does inform providers on whether or not the service member they are treating would benefit from proactive, early intervention and treatment to limit future injuries and illnesses in areas AI has identified.

While the goal of the MERIT project is to keep our service members at the ready for their military roles, it has broad applications in civilian healthcare. As my colleague Michelle Padgett of the JAIC's Warfighter Health Team says, "We have an opportunity to change the landscape for healthcare delivery. This requires an evolution from current program and product-thinking to an ecosystem of shared data and services. AI in healthcare presents a wholesale shift from where we are today, benefiting health and our nation."

We all know that healthcare providers today usually don't have time to sit and chat with patients long enough to get a full grasp of all the factors impacting their current conditions. The MERIT project and other AI initiatives can enable providers to get a full grasp not only of the patient's medical history but also of predicted health issues in seconds. Before we make a clinical decision, AI can scan and consider the patient's entire record. As the article says, "The real value of AI is the speed in which it can process huge amounts of data to give a holistic view of the service member that enables the medical provider to use their time effectively with the service member. These AI capabilities can operate around the clock, much like a "Check Engine Light" in your vehicle, continually scanning medical records to alert medical providers when an intervention (checkup) is needed."

In Houston, Texas, Memorial Hermann Health System used AI's ability to facilitate data management to solve a different problem. Despite years of training and education programs, providers were still not documenting all the diagnoses being managed in acute care patients. Now, AI takes a comprehensive look at patients' charts, ensures that the documentation reflects the care provided, and prompts providers to fully enter diagnoses.

Courage to Face the Future

Maya Angelou once said, "One isn't necessarily born with courage, but one is born with potential. Without courage, we cannot practice any other virtue with consistency. We can't be kind, true, merciful, generous, or honest." With this statement, she delivered the essential wisdom of the necessary ingredient of courage we all need in order to make a positive difference in our world.

Regardless of your past, present, or perceived future, you have the potential to be courageous. Leaving an impact on the world just requires courage. So many brilliant ideas and life-altering breakthroughs are withheld because of a lack of courage. The only way you will leave an imprint in the wrinkles of time is to constantly take steps. Employ courage and trod out a path all your own. The life you have been blessed with will only be lived once. You are the star of your own motion picture, and every moment is a new scene. And it is being shot digitally.

Pandemics, politics, wars, hunger—today's world can be a frightening place. Letting go of what we know, what we're comfortable with, and what we once expected from the rest of our lives and our practice of healthcare can be frightening. But there is a new future waiting for us. A new future in medicine—a future helped along by AI.

The impact you leave on the world will be a combination of your courage, your capacity to love, and your willingness to go against the grain—including the grain of your own expectations. Therefore, do it. Have courage, spread love, dare to make an impact, and don't hesitate to do it in ways you haven't considered before.

AI expands the *purpose* of healthcare from simply healing to supporting wellness that predicts and prevents new health issues before they arise. AI can help you *personalize* the time you spend with patients or clients, creating meaningful encounters where you can really get to know the people you serve. AI also expands the *partnership* that providers, health systems, and payors can build as we access a global network of resources available in a click.

AI Changing Lives

Congressional Report on AI

"America is not prepared to defend or compete in AI era." Investments in talent, research, development and manufacturing are needed now to *"build the best tools the fastest and know how to use them."* The report says AI has *"immense potential both to help and to hurt."* Let's invest in AI as a human care helper and tool for democracy.

FIVE AI Lessons Learned from Finishing 21 Marathons

If you want to learn about yourself, run a marathon. If you want to learn about life, run more than one. On September 13, 2020, amid the COVID-19 pandemic, I finished my twenty-first marathon (virtually), the 124th Boston Marathon. During my 26.2-mile journey, I learned about myself, reflected on my AI journey, and learned even more about life. Only a year prior, I embarked on a new assignment in a new role to leverage AI and deliver improved capability to those who care for warfighters. Indeed, the task was a natural extension of my work as a physician and surgeon.

Regrettably, the pandemic made an already difficult job more challenging. Separated from my team and forced to have virtual meetings added a unique dimension of stress, and on many occasions I seriously doubted we would make any progress. On the way to completing my twenty-first marathon, I thought about five AI lessons I have learned over the years.

1. **Don't be afraid to start.** *The 124th Boston Marathon, initially scheduled for Patriot's Day, April 20, 2020, was postponed multiple times and canceled before a virtual event was eventually sanctioned. I was ill-prepared, feeling less than optimally fit and anxious. I was afraid to start and considered packing it in rather than face the 26.2 miles of uncertainty. Fortunately, I overcame my fear and stepped out into my neighborhood with a vague plan of how I would cover the distance. Ultimately, starting the virtual race was a good decision. I discovered things I never noticed before.*

   Working with AI is also full of new beginnings, and each transition can be very intimidating. The beginning of an endeavor, relationship, or business requires facing uncertainty. When you overcome fear and start on the AI journey, you will discover things you never noticed before. For example, we at the JAIC learned that many of our legacy systems were not capable of supporting machine learning. Our computer power was woefully insufficient, and our cloud storage capacity was inadequate to scale. An entirely new strategy for infrastructure modernization was necessary.

2. **Never underestimate your team's potential.** *My marathon story started with a bet. In 2002, after a spirited debate with*

a surgical colleague about the upcoming 2004 Olympics, we
made a gentleman's bet of $1 on whether or not I could finish
a marathon (although I was never a runner). I entered and
"won" the lottery for the 2003 New York City Marathon. With
little background in distance running, I read everything about
marathons and followed the sage advice of one marathoner:
"Drive 26.2 miles so you respect the distance." I drove 26.2
miles. Wow! What a distance to cover running. Over a few
months, I followed instructions in the books, increased daily
running, talked to other runners and especially marathoners
about training for and running a marathon, and learned much.

In life, reading books, especially about a brand-new subject
like AI, can bring great insight and provide a virtual road map
for how to navigate what seems impossible at first. Meeting
with AI experts was especially rewarding. As we worked on
AI projects, I began to understand more about the subject.
Combining that knowledge with the practical application of
developing AI solutions with a talented team proved to be a
winning strategy. After driving those 26.2 intimidating miles,
I could never imagine I would now have a running resume that
includes twenty-one finishes, including Boston (2020). I won the
bet, still have my dollar, and applied the lessons learned to my
work in AI.

3. **You will always get what you want in life if you help
others.** *After completing my first marathon, I caught "marathon*
fever." I wanted to run more marathons. Each race brought

new goals. I aimed to run faster, and in some marathons, I did improve. Yet in others, I was slower despite arduous training. It was frustrating. Like many serious marathoners, qualifying for the Boston Marathon was my Holy Grail. For years, a Boston qualifying time was elusive, and as I aged, it rapidly faded to the realm of impossibility.

Then, in 2016, after a challenging overseas military deployment and a long marathon hiatus, an opportunity to run the Boston Marathon as a charity runner emerged. By serving and helping others, I was able to fulfill a dream. Now, four Boston Marathons later, I have learned how important the lesson of service is to AI work. As the JAIC helped deliver AI capabilities to our stakeholders, we engendered support from others who returned in kind and further advanced our progress.

4. **It is not magic that makes it work; it's the work that makes the magic.** *The Disney Marathon in Orlando, Florida, was, by far, my slowest marathon ever. My run was interrupted along the way to visit with the characters, and I was enamored, like most children, by Disney's spectacle. I learned about all the work it takes to "make the magic happen." So much work goes on behind the scenes and when the show begins, you quickly forget how it all happened.*

This lesson was never lost to me with our work in AI. We realized how hard it was to curate data, prepare and label data, and make that data amenable to machine learning—not to mention the necessary work of talented engineers building infrastructure and dedicated data scientists who enabled code to perform magic. Running a marathon is the same way. It takes a lot of work to arrive at the start line of a marathon, and when the show begins, it may look easy as you cover the distance, especially for the elite runners. But when you look behind the scenes, you realize the great ones train every day, all year long, endlessly, for hours and hours. It takes work—hard work—to make AI magic come to life.

5. **Put one foot in front of the other. Repeat.** *This simple lesson is so relevant for the marathon and essential for creating successful AI solutions in healthcare and in life. In the course of 26.2 miles, so much can and will go wrong. In all my marathons, I began with a plan. It was a plan for my pace, a method for my stride, a plan for how and when I would fuel and hydrate my body, and even a plan for how I would cope when my plan failed. Despite all my planning, in every marathon, my careful plan rarely survived contact with the brutal reality of those formidable 26.2 miles. My 2020 virtual Boston Marathon was no exception. It was the first time I attempted to cover that distance virtually (without the support of cheering crowds and other runners), and none of my other marathons could prepare me for this one.*

It was the same for our virtual AI work during the pandemic. None of our teams' previous experience could quite prepare us for what we encountered. Yet we pushed on and became very effective. Like the marathoner, we relied on a tried-and-true axiom. Put one foot in front of the other, and repeat.

When we were in doubt, and doubt occurred frequently, we put one foot in front of the other and repeated until we crossed the finish line for each of the outlined goals. Many plans are abandoned in the uncertainty that characterizes the human condition of loss, grief, triumph, and redemption in life.

In those uncertain times, especially when faced with the difficult task of introducing a new order through AI, the best way to proceed is to put one foot in front of the other, despite all the pain, and repeat. A finish line and better tomorrow will eventually be on the horizon.

AI Changing Lives

Are You Ready to Collaborate With AI?

You better be! The use of AI at scale will add as much as $15.7 trillion to the global economy by 2030. AI changes how companies work and who does the work.

Afterword

Severence M. MacLaughlin, PhD
Founder, DeLorean Artificial Intelligence

I sometimes struggle to communicate what I do to those closest to me. My mother often asks, "What do you actually do? I am trying to explain your technologies to my friends." I love references to popular culture and explained my AI to my mum. "Mah, have you seen *The Terminator*?" "Yes, with Arnold, right?" my mum responded. "I am building Skynet, but the caring pink bunny rabbit version."

I will send *The Art of Human Care with AI* to my mother! I love this book. Dr. Hassan Tetteh breaks down what artificial intelligence is, demystifies it, and explains the current and future potential of this potent network of developing technologies as it is applied to healthcare. Dr. Tetteh accomplished what I have failed to do over the past ten years—he can explain what AI is to my mum!

Be thankful Dr. Tetteh is a physician leader within the military, caring for our nation's most important treasure, our troops and veterans. His kind, empathetic, adept understanding of new technology and how to apply it to care for those injured and sick is refreshing. Dr. Tetteh is the type of physician I pray will care for my mum and family when needed.

Dr. Tetteh points out that AI is *not* futuristic. AI is happening now and evolving daily. The COVID-19 pandemic has advanced a global digital transformation by years and concomitantly accelerated the implementation and adoption of AI in healthcare. Why? Because we had to. The pandemic was, for some, an evolutionary or extinction event. The organizations that were prepared to change and evolve established the infrastructure for AI and were ready to deploy.

The amount of available data has doubled since data started being collected. By 2025 the vast amount of available data is expected to double annually. Why is this important? With such an exponential increase in available data, there is no way for humans to comb through this treasure trove to understand the knowledge that could be unlocked. Dr. Tetteh describes this as finding a "golden needle" in a haystack—golden because of the similar color to the hay but also the value of the needle once it is found. When you or a loved one requires medical attention, you want your physician to have all the available data and information possible to make better and informed decisions for your medical treatment.

Imagine your doctor having access to every physician and how they treated a patient with similar symptoms—now that is power. Imagine your doctor walking into your treatment room when you are the most vulnerable with an iPad or tablet that is connected to an AI persona that has analyzed all of your vitals, diagnostics, and symptoms and compared that to millions of others and has recommended to the doctor a hyper-personalized treatment plan based on billions of data points. AI's power in the healthcare field is arming our healthcare professionals with unparalleled information and predicting how a patient will respond to treatment. Imagine delaying dialysis for a kidney patient for six months, predicting the onset of COPD or diabetes, and what to do to prevent it. AI's power brings better healthcare, a better quality of life, and more time with those we love.

The description of AI assisting physicians and health plans to deliver the best quality care in real time is not a futuristic event. It is happening now. Healthcare organizations and government bodies are investing to drive improved health outcomes and decrease costs and waste. One of the challenges to bring the vision that Dr. Tetteh has so eloquently described is access to healthcare data. Currently in the United States, the majority of healthcare data does not reside with physicians. Still, the healthcare payers may be insurance companies or government agencies such as the Centers for Medicare & Medicaid Services (CMS), Veterans Affairs (VA), or the Defense Health Agency (DHA). These organizations are working diligently to share data and promote electronic health record interoperability. Why is this important? Having an extensive, unified data set for millions of patients allows for the analysis of treatment pathways, which allows for the prediction of the best course of treatment. If we had this unified data source and sharing capability during the COVID-19 pandemic, we as a nation would have been able to treat the infections faster and more efficiently, knowing what treatment modalities work best for different patient populations.

We should all be thankful for the thoughtful, compassionate, curious, and innovative individuals who led the way for AI innovation in the federal government and civilian sectors. As Dr. Tetteh describes in this book, the military has historically been instrumental in advancing medical technologies over the years and will lead again. The DOD, DHA, VA, Centers for Disease Control and Prevention (CDC), and CMS curate vast amounts of health information, which will fuel evolving AI technologies in healthcare. As Dr. Tetteh espouses, these organizations and others could employ the human care tenets of purpose, personalization, and partnerships to achieve an impactful and positive healthcare revolution through AI.

We are at an exciting time in the field of AI science and medicine. We need to educate our fellow citizens on AI's power and how it will impact our health. To that end, Dr. Tetteh has engendered a fresh, creative vision and advanced the conversation with this book. Scientists need to communicate "the art of the possible" and continually improve our scientific process. Collectively, we have the elements and potential, as outlined in *The Art of Human Care with AI,* to work toward a better, brighter healthcare future with AI.

acknowledgments

This book would not exist without the service, care, sacrifice, and compassion of all who have cared for another human. I am incredibly thankful to those who work every day in our places of healing to do the hard work of restoring health and wellness and the innovators that bring us new technology to do our work better. These individuals deserve all the honor.

I am indebted to the many patients I met over the years, for they provided inspiration and wisdom. Stories and drama connect more effectively with people than facts and random words. Thus, Nikias and Hippocrates's story were adapted from a book called *The Sublime Engine: A Biography of the Human Heart* by brothers Stephen and Thomas Amidon. Tom Siebel's *Digital Transformation: Survive and Thrive in an Era of Mass Extinction* provided invaluable context to characterize AI and healthcare for the present day. Special thanks to my research advisors and mentors at the National War College, Kelly Ward, John Via, and John W. Yaeger. Additionally, thanks to Mark Beckner, Margo Edmunds, Eric Elster, Andy Gettinger, Matt Goldman, Caesar Junker, Ryan Kappadel,

Arthur Kellerman, Rebecca Lee, Danyelle Long, Michael Malanoski, Scott McKeithen, Nand Mulchandani, Chris Nichols, Niels Olson, Michelle Padgett, Jeremy Pamplin, Andrew Plummer, Charles Rice, Adam Robinson, Pete Walker, and Jonathan Woodson for their invaluable contributions and for sharing their thoughts and perspectives on AI and medicine.

My teachers, mentors, and coaches have directly and indirectly influenced this work and taught me the healing art of medicine. The conceptual, editorial, and artistic support of Jack Canfield, Colin Carroll, Steven Dana, Bettina Experton, Rose Freeman, Doug Fridsma, Lieutenant General Michael S. Groen, Severence MacLaughlin, Karen McDiarmid, Thomas Moran, Keith Salzman, Estelle Slootmaker, Stoney Trent, Lieutenant General (Retired) John 'Jack' Shanahan, and James Tessier was priceless.

Finally, the most thanks must go to my family, especially my wife Lisa, son Edmund, and daughter Ella, to tolerate and support both a surgeon's and an author's schedule. Thank you all for always listening at the kitchen table to endless recitals, for enduring many drafts and revisions, and for your patience, love, and support with tea, a special treat, and warm embrace through many days and long nights. You are all a blessing. I am fortunate to have and thank God for every day.

Hic Pro Bonus
Here for Good...

Hassan A. Tetteh MD
Washington, D.C.

References

Hippocrates (2012). *Hippocrates aphorismi* (Latin edition). San Bernardino, CA: Ulan Press.

Amidon, S., and Amidon, T. (2011). *The sublime engine: A biography of the human heart.* Emmaus, PA: Rodale Books.

Baldwin, R. (2016). *The great convergence.* Cambridge, MA: Harvard University Press.

Daugherty, P. R., and Wilson, H. J. (2018). *Human + machine: Reimagining work in the age of AI.* Cambridge, MA: Harvard Business Review Press.

Lohr, S. (2015). *Data-ism.* New York: Harper Collins Publishers.

Newport, C. (2016). *Deep work: Rules for success in a distracted world.* New York: Grand Central Press.

Nadella, S. (2017). *Hit refresh: The quest to rediscover Microsoft's soul and imagine a better future for everyone.* New York: Harper Collins.

Taleb, N. N. (2010). *Black swan: The impact of the highly improbable.* New York: Random House.

Tegmark, M. (2017). *Life 3.0: Being human in the age of artificial intelligence.* New York: Alfred A. Knopf.

Tetteh, H. (2018). *Artificial intelligence and military medicine: Strategic application of the technology of our era* [Master's thesis]. National Defense University, National War College.

About the Author

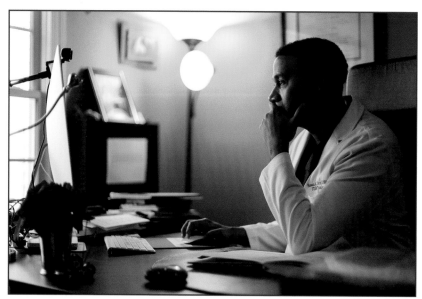

Photo by Angela Vasquez

DR. HASSAN A. TETTEH is a U.S. Navy Captain
and Associate Professor of Surgery at the Uniformed Services
University of the Health Sciences and adjunct faculty at Howard
University College of Medicine. He was selected a 2019 Emerging
Leader in Health and Medicine Scholar by the National Academy
of Medicine. Currently, Tetteh is a Thoracic Surgeon for MedStar
Health and Walter Reed National Military Medical Center. He
leads a Specialized Thoracic Adapted Recovery (STAR) Team in
Washington, DC, and his research in thoracic transplantation aims
to expand heart and lung recovery and save lives.

A native of Brooklyn, New York, Tetteh received his BS from State University of New York (SUNY) at Plattsburgh, his MD from SUNY Downstate Medical Center, his MPA from Harvard's Kennedy School of Government, an MBA from Johns Hopkins University Carey Business School, and an MS in National Security Strategy with a concentration in Artificial Intelligence from the National War College. He completed his thoracic surgery fellowship at the University of Minnesota and his advanced cardiac surgery fellowship at Harvard Medical School's Brigham and Women's Hospital in Boston.

Tetteh is the founder and principal of Tetteh Consulting Group, the creator of *The Art of Human Care* book series, and a best-selling author of several books, including *Gifts of the Heart, Star Patrol,* and *The Art of Human Care.* Tetteh is board certified in thoracic surgery, general surgery, clinical informatics, and healthcare management, and is a Fellow of the American College of Surgeons, a Fellow of the American College of Healthcare Executives, and a Fellow of the American Medical Informatics Association.

Tetteh received the Alley Sheridan Award from the Thoracic Surgery Foundation for Research and Education, was named a TEDMED Front Line Scholar, and is a TEDx speaker. He's an alumnus of the Harvard Medical School Writers' Workshop and the Yale Writers' Conference and lives near Washington, DC, with his wife, son, and daughter.

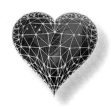

KUdOS

"An amazing journey from a brilliant mind! Dr. Tetteh reminds us what it means to be human and challenges us to find our purpose and have the courage to make the art of the possible a reality."

Kevin A. Dorrance, MD, FACP, Partner and CEO TransformCare

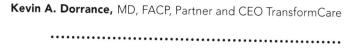

"Dr. Tetteh provides impactful insight of AI's potential and role in the Art of Human Care. It is a must read for anyone who wants to better understand and improve the application of AI in medicine but more importantly in caring for the whole person."

Paul A. Gurny, Senior Professional Faculty at Johns Hopkins University

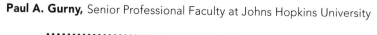

"Dr. Tetteh is a true polymath. The perspective he brings—as a clinician, a military officer, an information scientist, and a humanitarian—enriches everything he does. And now, he brings that perspective to consider how healthcare, what he calls "human care," can be vastly improved through the application of artificial intelligence. At first, this looks like an oxymoron; from all the science fiction we have seen and read, "human" and "AI" seem diametrically opposed. Yet, Dr. Tetteh explains—with passion and logic—how AI can accelerate advances in healthcare. Perhaps AI is not "Dr. Tetteh's Magic Bullet," but it can certainly improve the human condition."

Douglas E. Hough, Ph.D., Senior Associate, Department of Health Policy and Management, Johns Hopkins University Bloomberg School of Public Health

"*The Art of Human Care with AI* is a compelling read for those of us who may not be AI experts but are trying to reshape healthcare for the better. Dr. Tetteh is one of those unique and rare individuals who has the credibility and experience to speak to both aspects of healthcare and the impact of AI on the future of health."

Joseph Shepherd Miller, Esq, Technology & Media Law & Policy Attorney, Founder of Washington Center for Technology Policy Inclusion, WashingTECH, Inc.